Skills that Build Confidence.
Data that Proves Impact.

DIGITAL HEALTH: ONE CLICK AT A TIME

WORKBOOK

By Angela Harris

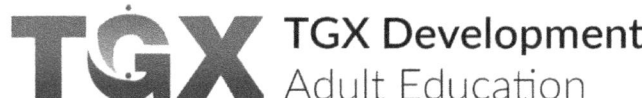

Digital Health: One Click at a Time

© 2025 TGX Development, LLC

Published by TGX Development, LLC
P.O. Box 14214
Research Triangle Park, NC 27709
Email: info@tgxdevelopment.com
Website: www.tgxdevelopment.com

ALL RIGHTS RESERVED. No part of this publication may be reproduced, stored in a retrieval system or transmitted, in any form or by any means, electronic, mechanical, photocopying, recording or otherwise, without the prior written permission of the publisher.

Trademarks: CLEAR Head Approach, CLEAR Framework, Howie's How-Tos, Sugaroo, Tech-for-Care Advocate, and The R.E.E.L. are trademarks of TGX Development. All other trademarks are the property of their respective owners. TGX Development is not associated with any product or vendor mentioned in this book.

Limit of Liability/Disclaimer of Warranty: While the publisher and author have used their best efforts in preparing this book, they make no representations or warranties with respect to the accuracy or completeness of the contents and specifically disclaim any implied warranties of merchantability or fitness for a particular purpose. The information, advice, and strategies contained herein are for educational purposes only and may not be suitable for your situation. Readers should consult with qualified health or other professionals where appropriate.

Further, readers should be aware that websites listed in this work may have changed or become unavailable between when this work was written and when it is read. Neither the publisher nor the author shall be liable for any loss, injury, or damages — including, but not limited to, personal, health-related, special, incidental, consequential, or commercial damages.

Digital Health: One Click at a Time
ISBN 979-8-9906801-2-8

For permission to use material from this text or product, email:
service@tgxdevelopment.com

For special premiums and sales promotions, email:
sales@tgxdevelopment.com

Printed in the United States of America

Digital Health: One Click at a Time

TABLE OF CONTENTS

ABOUT THIS BOOK 4

LESSON ONE: What is Digital Health? 5
Digital Health Overview 6
Examples of Digital Health 8
The R.E.E.L: Circle of Care 11
Moving to a Paperless Environment 14
Howie's How-Tos: Preparing for
  Paperless Care 17
Artificial Intelligence and Care 21
Key Terms 26

LESSON TWO: Online Patient Portals 28
Getting Started 29
The R.E.E.L: Patient Portal Login Page 30
Inside the Portal 32
Howie's How-Tos: Friends and Family
  Access 34
Preventive Screenings 37
Key Terms 39

LESSON THREE: Telehealth Visits 40
Online Scheduling 41
Preparing for Your Visit 44
Using Generative AI 44
The R.E.E.L: Tech-for-Care Advocate 46
Checking In 47
Key Terms 50

LESSON FOUR: Everyday Care 51
Mobile Health Apps 52
Howie's How-Tos: Finding and Using
  Health Apps 54
Remote Patient Monitoring 57
The R.E.E.L: Aging in Place 60
Key Terms 62

**LESSON FIVE: Trusting Health
  Information** 63
Health Misinformation 64

Howie's How-Tos: Spotting Fear and
  Propaganda 65
CLEAR Head Approach 68
AI for Fact-Finding 71
The R.E.E.L: Voice Use for
  AI Fact-Finding 74
Key Terms 76

**LESSON SIX: Protecting Health
  Information** 77
Patient Rights 78
Patient Responsibilities 82
Suspicious Emails 82
Two-Factor Authentication 84
The R.E.E.L: Healthcare Fraud 85
Keeping Care Safe 87
Key Terms 90

**LESSON SEVEN: Working with Your
  Care Team** 91
Teaming Up for Positive Outcomes 92
Feedback to Improve Care 95
Practice Survey 96
Partnering Across Digital Health Skills 99
The R.E.E.L: Speaking Up 100
Key Terms 102

ACKNOWLEDGMENTS 103
ABOUT THE AUTHOR 103
ENDNOTES 104
ANSWER KEYS 105
Lesson One 106
Lesson Two 113
Lesson Three 117
Lesson Four 120
Lesson Five 125
Lesson Six 129
Lesson Seven 134

Building Skills, Tracking Progress, Improving Care

This workbook is part of the **Tech-for-Care Advocate™ system**, designed to help adult educators strengthen digital health skills, improve care, and demonstrate measurable impact. Each lesson builds confidence in using patient portals, telehealth, health apps, and artificial intelligence (AI) tools — aligned to the **National Health Education Standards** and informed by research and insights from leading **healthcare practitioners, health technology experts,** and **insurance payers.** The workbook also supports classroom-to-career pathways by building digital, health literacy, and critical thinking skills essential for today's health-related roles.

By activating your site's **checkpoint system** (via the QR code below), you'll gain more than a curriculum. You'll unlock a simple, data-driven tool that tracks learner growth, builds accountability, and supports continuous program improvement without extra software.

Supporting Learning and Accountability

The checkpoint system includes:
- **Pre- and post-checkpoint links** for each lesson
- **Site-level data** on learner confidence, understanding, and intent to apply skills
- **Exportable summaries** to support grants, reports, and instructional planning

Each lesson also includes **clear objectives, key health terms,** and **practice activities** that make digital health skills **practical, relevant, and immediately applicable** — strengthening trust across the circle of care and helping learners actively participate in their own care.

Getting started takes less than 2 minutes.

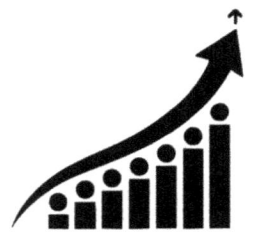

Turn learning into measurable outcomes. Scan the QR code to begin checkpoints and reporting. (Available only to registered sites.)

LESSON ONE: What is Digital Health?

Introduction

Objectives – After completing this lesson, you will be able to:

- Describe your circle of care
- Connect digital health terms to real people and services you recognize
- Identify examples of digital health
- Choose the right place of care based on the situation
- Explain what it's like to receive care in a paperless environment
- Understand how the use of mobile health apps achieves care goals
- Engage artificial intelligence to obtain health information

Key Terms

- AI Prompt
- Artificial Intelligence
- Chatbot
- Circle of Care
- Data
- Dietary Supplement
- Digital Health
- Electronic Health Record (EHR)
- Electronic Prescription
- Electronic Signature
- E-Visit
- Health Insurance
- Hydration
- In-Network
- Medicaid
- Medicare
- Medication
- Mobile Health App
- Over-the-Counter
- Patient Portal
- Prescription Drug
- Telehealth
- Telemedicine
- Video Call
- Virtual Reality
- Wearable Device

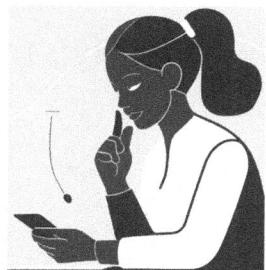

Let's Get Started!

Your voice matters. Enter your site code and the information below to share what you already know and what you hope to learn about digital health.

| Lesson One | Checkpoint Number: **1** |

Digital Health Overview

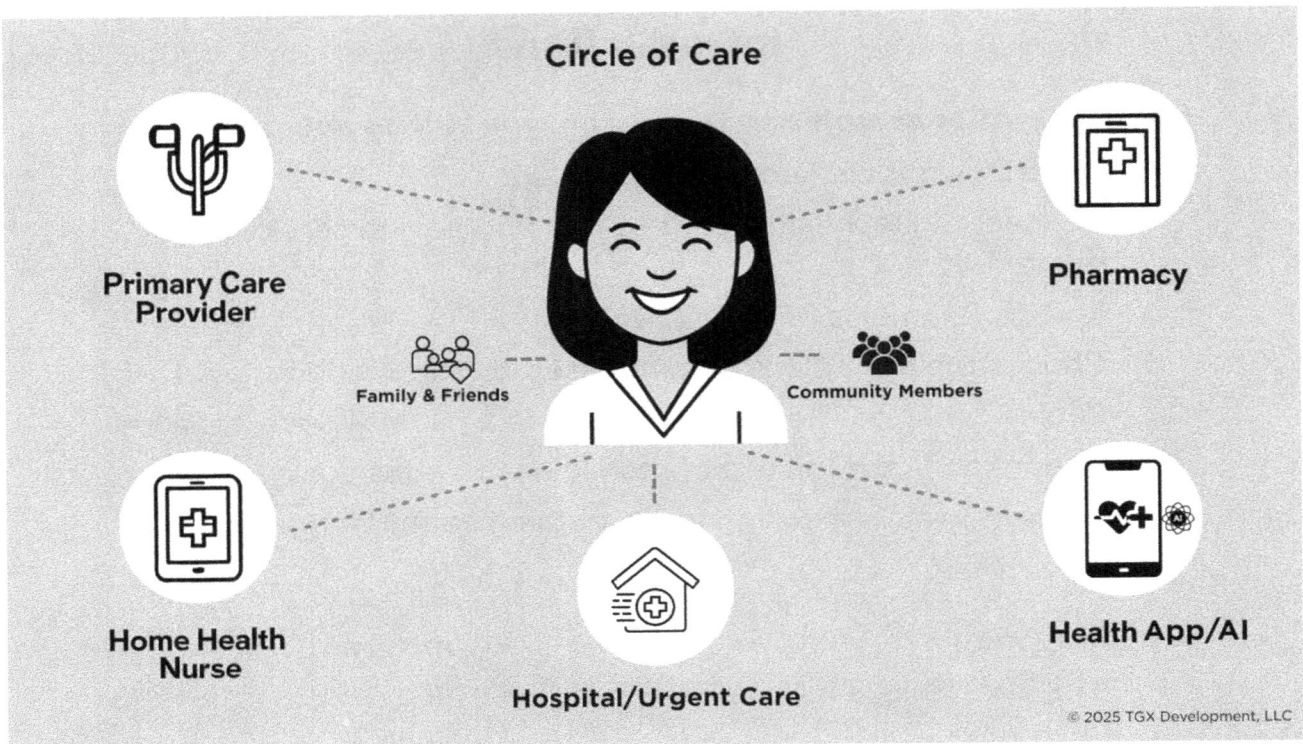

Have you thought about the people and places in your **circle of care**? Technology is now creating a support system that connects you with people, places, and your health information, shaping how you engage with and interact with healthcare.

Digital health means using technology like phones, computers, or apps to take care of your health, talk to your doctor, get medicine, and learn how to stay healthy, while keeping your personal health information safe. It helps identify and connect individuals in your circle of care so that you have an improved health journey. Your circle of care might include different doctors, some family members, a nurse who helps at home, a physical therapist, and someone who helps translate or explain medical information. Digital health helps these people work as a team by letting them see the same care information online, if you say it is okay, so they can support you better.

Digital health brings many benefits, but there are also some important things to watch out for when using it.

Benefits of Digital Health:

- **It helps you see a doctor without leaving home.**
  You can have video visits or send messages using a computer or phone.

- **You can check your health anytime.**
  Apps and devices can show your steps, heart rate, or remind you to take medicine.

- **It makes getting help faster.**
  You don't have to wait in long lines or be placed on hold, listening to music or automated messages until someone, or a **chatbot**, becomes available to assist you. <u>Note:</u> A chatbot is a virtual assistant that uses artificial intelligence to answer your questions, help you access healthcare information, and connect you with the right medical professional.

- **It helps you learn more about your health.**
  You can read tips, answer questions with personalized answers, or watch videos to stay healthy and understand your body better.

- **It keeps your health information safe in one place.**
  You can log in to a private account to see all your medical records when you need them.

Reasons to Be Careful:

- **Your health information is private.**
  You don't want the wrong people to see your personal health records.

- **Some websites or apps might not be safe.**
  Not every health tool online is real or helpful.

- **Scams can happen.**
  Some people try to trick others into giving away personal or financial information.

- **It's easy to get confused.**
  Health words and tools can be hard to understand without help.

- **Not all information online is true.**
  Just because something is on the internet doesn't mean it is right for your health. When in doubt, consult a trusted healthcare professional.

Examples of Digital Health

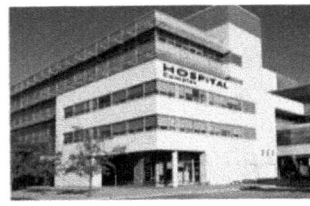 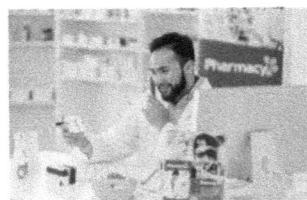 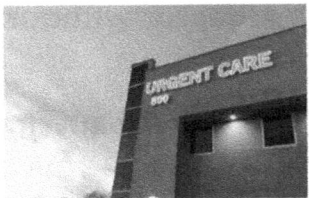 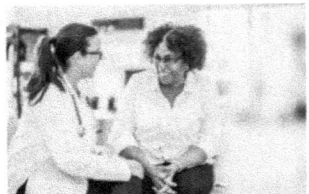

Traditional Places of Care

Technology is expanding the places of care. Years ago places of care were limited to hospitals, pharmacies, clinics, and the doctor's office. Today, technology makes it possible to administer care and promote wellbeing in spaces not confined to traditional places of care. Having an internet connection and secure ways of sending and receiving information have created environments where health can be managed in innovative ways. Technology-enabled methods of care include e-visits, video calls, wearable devices, and virtual reality.

Christopher is engaged in an **e-visit,** which is a way to safely give and receive information about his health virtually, without interacting with an individual directly. In this instance he is using a **patient portal**, which is a secure website or app that lets users review their health information, including test results, upcoming appointments, and messages from their doctor. Patients can also communicate with their doctor and schedule their own appointments.

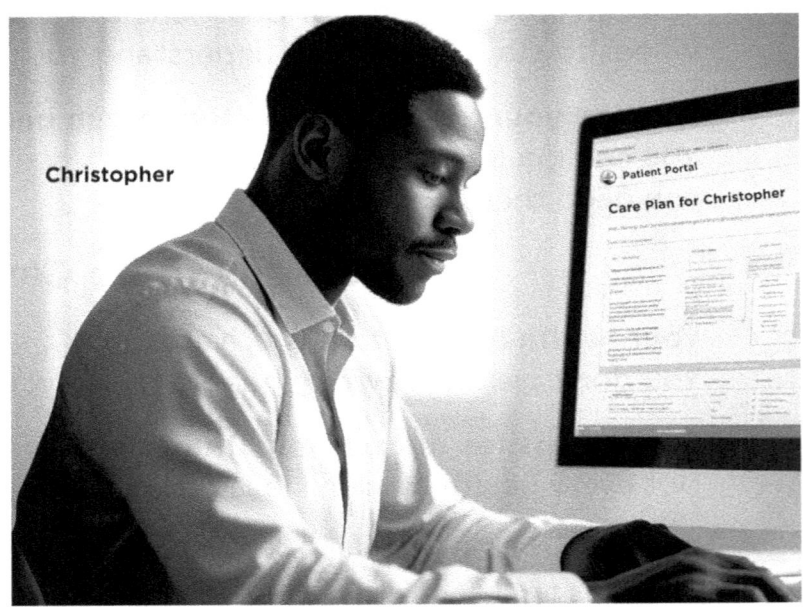

E-Visit

E-Visits can be suitable for the following situations:

- Minor health concerns like a cold, cough, heartburn, or sinus issue.
- Simple skin conditions like a rash, acne, or insect bite, especially when you have a photo that can be shared with your doctor.
- Medication adjustments or prescription refills.
- Non-urgent matters that do not require face-to-face interactions.

Caroline is having a **video call**, or live virtual visit, with her doctor. She is using a safe app that her care provider helped her get from her patient portal. With fast internet and the camera on her laptop, she can talk to her doctor from home in a private and comfortable setting.

A video call is generally appropriate for the following situations:

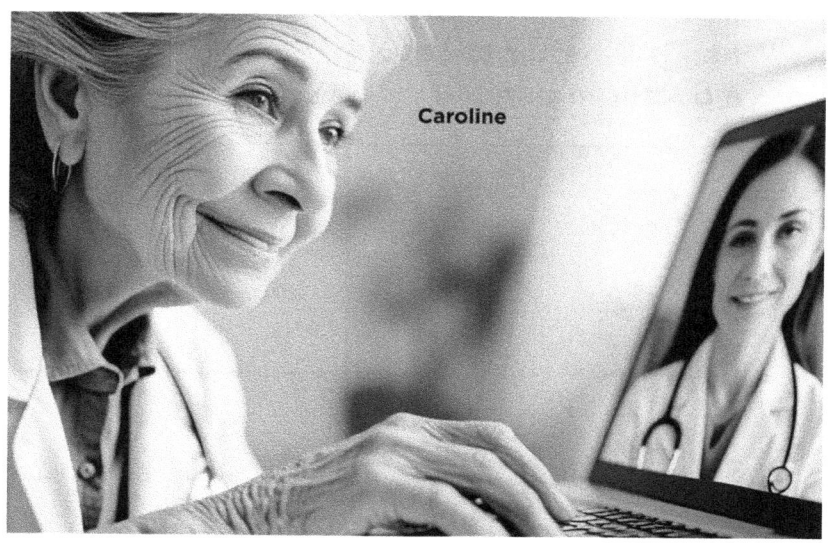
Video Call

- A follow-up visit to discuss progress and concerns regarding an ongoing medical condition like diabetes or arthritis.
- Mental health support.
- Speaking with your doctor about lab tests or X-ray results.

When is it better to see a doctor in person?	Situation
	You are experiencing stomach pain or have difficulty breathing and need a physical exam.
	You injure your ankle during a sporting event and the ankle looks abnormal. You also feel severe pain when trying to walk.
	It is time for your annual physical exam or a routine check-up.

When is it better to see a doctor in person?	Situation
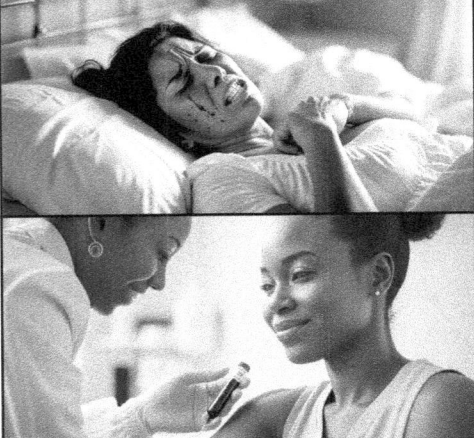	You are having a very serious emergency, like strong chest pain, trouble breathing, or bleeding that won't stop.
	You require an in-person lab test or other in-office procedure.

LeeAnn is using her smart watch to track her heart rate. This smart watch is a type of **wearable device**, which is connected to the internet and worn on the body. It can remind LeeAnn to get up and move or take her medicine. Other examples of a wearable device include a pair of glasses and a ring.

Virtual reality, which is a computer-made world that you can explore and interact with, also serves as a nontraditional way to improve healthcare. In the image featuring Kevin, virtual reality goggles help him practice physical therapy exercises in water. Kevin is able to see how to move and follow instructions to help his body heal in a real way, using a pretend place.

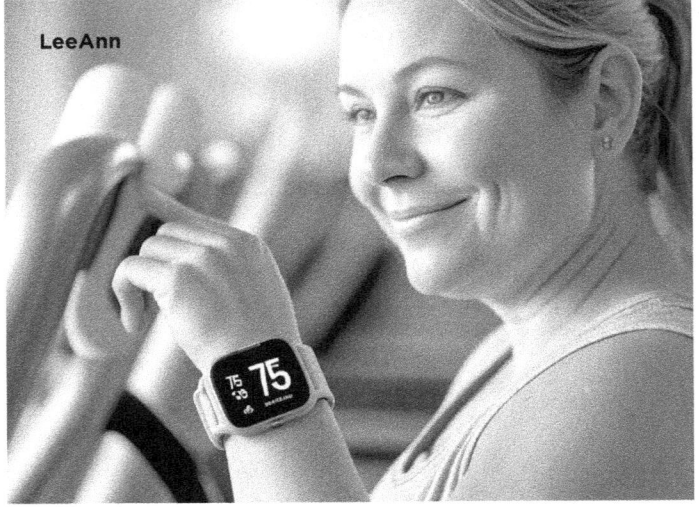
Wearable Device

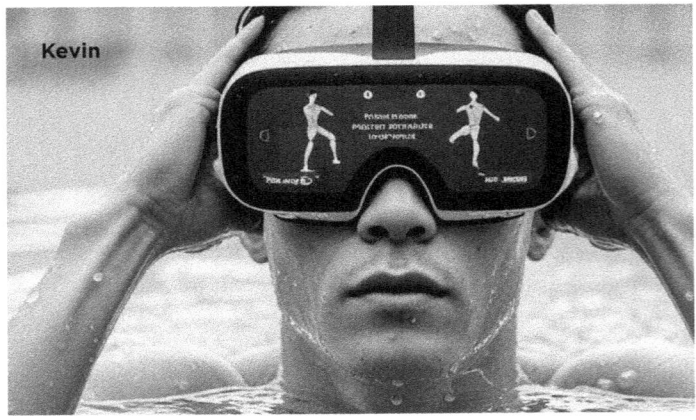
Virtual Reality

The R.E.E.L.

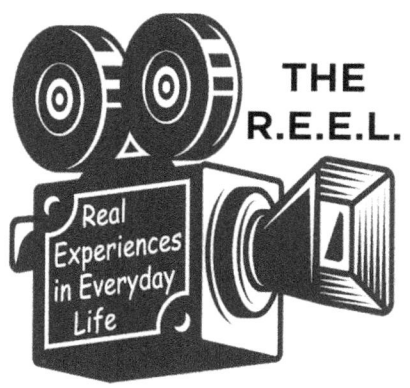

Circle of Care

Because healthy food, safe places to live, reliable transportation, and steady work are basic needs that affect a person's health, the circle of care is expanding to include a person's social environment.

Directions: Use the information in the passage and knowledge about your community to answer each question.

1. Who is in your circle of care?

   _____

   _____

2. Dana lives in another part of the country and is caring for her elderly mom who lives in **your community**. What resources are available to provide a hot meal or healthy food for Dana's mom who stays at home and is recovering from an illness?

   _____

   _____

3. When Dana's mom recovers and becomes active again, what resources are available in **your community** to ensure that she maintains her wellbeing and social connections?

   _____

   _____

   _____

Activity #1

Directions: It's time to check your understanding of digital health. Read each question. Circle the **best** answer.

1. When thinking about how people use technology for care, which answer best describes the **circle of care**?

    A) An online meeting place where doctors go to learn new skills.

    B) A team of people using digital tools to work together and give a person the care they need.

    C) The care team members shown in an individual's patient portal.

2. Susan's doctor has been treating her acne with a prescription medication. Susan just completed her last refill and now needs to request more of the same medication. Which of these places of care is the best choice to take care of Susan?

    A) Video call
    B) In-person visit
    C) E-Visit

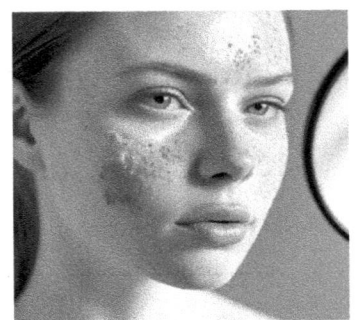

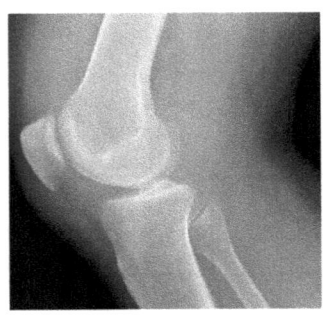

3. Victoria has received X-ray results regarding the arthritis in her right knee. She desires a follow-up visit with her doctor. Which of these places of care is the best choice for her follow-up visit?

    A) In-person visit
    B) E-Visit
    C) Video call

4. Larry twists his ankle during basketball practice and his coach tells him that it can be treated with rest, ice, compression, and elevation, also known as RICE. The coach further explains that RICE is a simple first-aid method used to treat sudden injuries like sprains, pulled muscles, and bruises. Which of these places of care is the best, immediate choice to take care of Larry?

    A) Rest at home
    B) Urgent care
    C) Video call

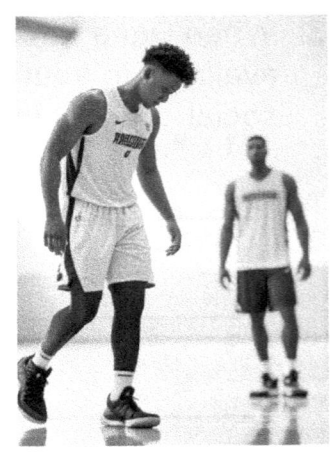

5. **True** or **False**. Write **T** for True or **F** for False next to the statements below.

_____ A) Digital health makes it less likely to be confused by unfamiliar health words and tools.

_____ B) Carter is wearing a ring that tracks his body temperature and sleep patterns. He is most likely wearing a smart ring, which is a type of wearable device.

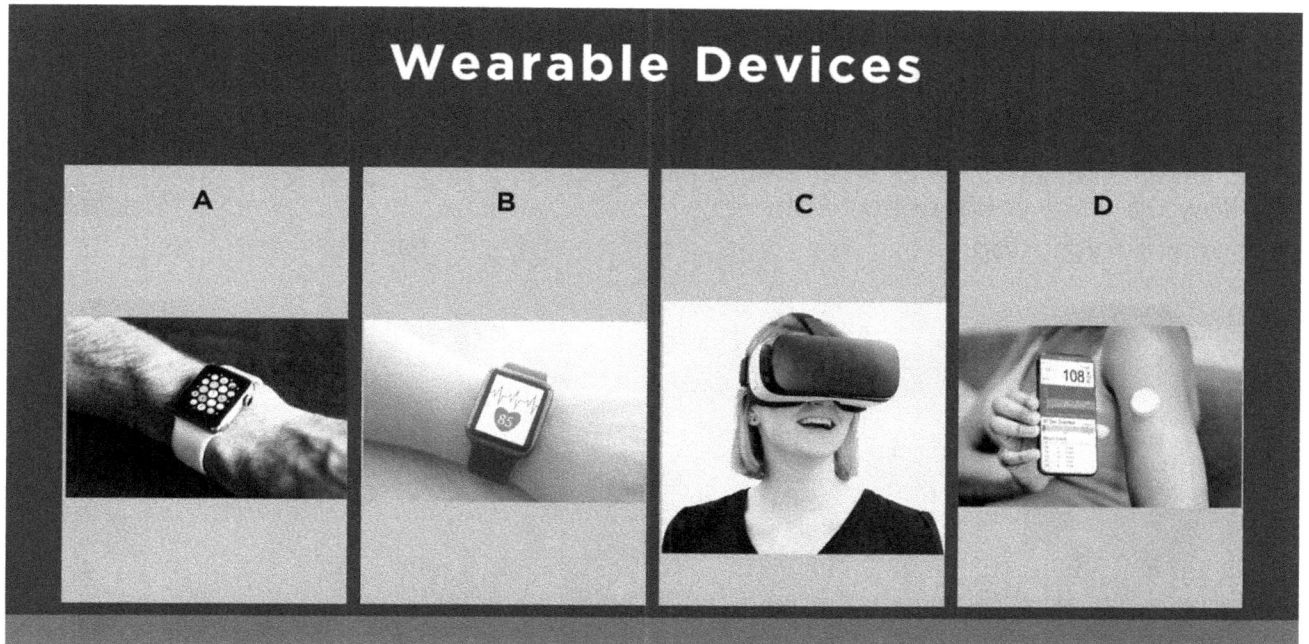

6. Now that you have seen some examples of wearable devices in the lesson, let's see if you can spot them on your own. Above are four pictures. Look at each one and identify the type of wearable device.

A) _____

B) _____

C) _____

D) _____

Moving to a Paperless Environment

We are quickly moving from the days of showing up at a doctor's office and filling out paperwork upon check-in. Many medical offices provide kiosks and tablets to make the process easier. Both kiosks and tablets have touchscreens that let you type in information without needing to talk to a staff member. Depending on whether you are visiting your doctor for the first time or going for a follow up visit, you'll need to share personal information.

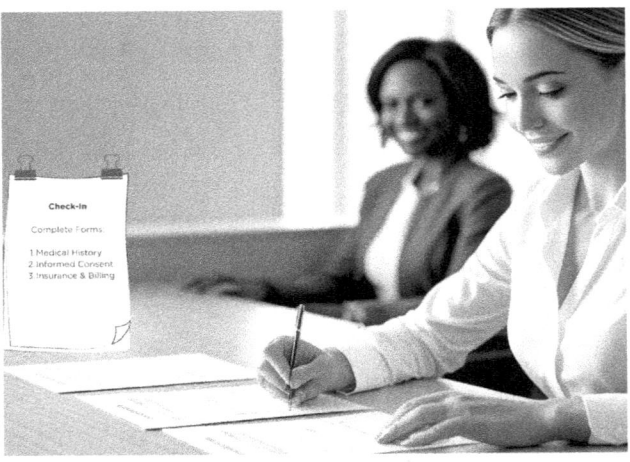

Paper Check-In

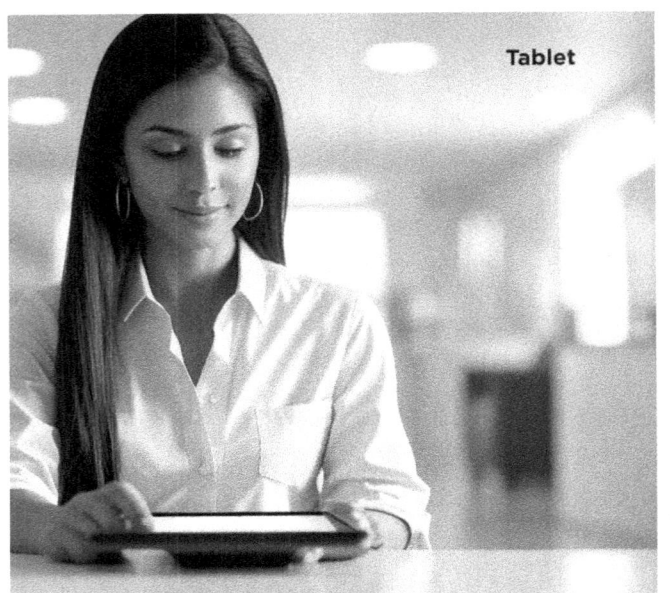
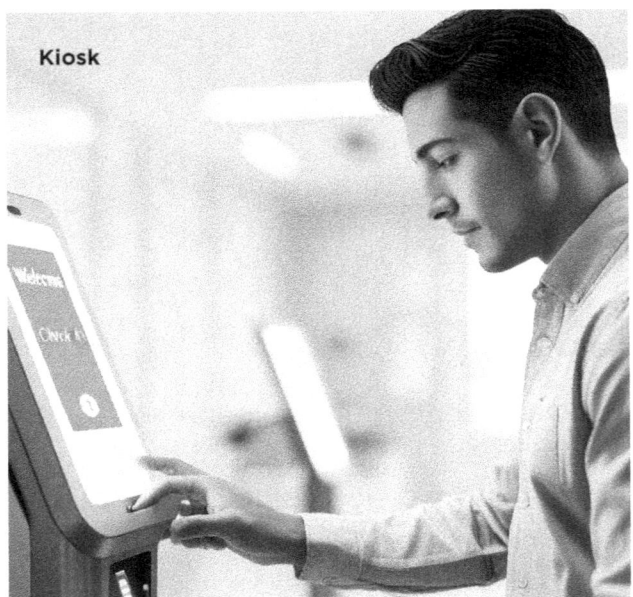

Paperless Check-In

This information will be added to a digital system and become part of your **electronic health record**. An electronic health record, sometimes referred to as an **EHR**, is a digital version of your medical history. It includes important health information like your medications, allergies, lab results, vaccinations, and treatment plans, and is stored on a computer instead of paper.

The following information supports check-in and represents the information often found in your electronic health record.

Personal	Insurance	Other
Name	Insurance Card	Reason for Visit
Date of Birth	Policy Number	Medications (Prescriptions and Dietary Supplements)
Contact Information (phone/email)	Group Number	Photo ID

Health insurance is a type of coverage that pays your medical bills when you get sick or injured. There are private insurance plans and government-sponsored plans like Medicare and Medicaid. Generally, **Medicare** is a federal health insurance program for people 65 years of age and older. **Medicaid**, on the other hand, provides coverage for low-income individuals and families. These forms of insurance cover doctor visits, hospital stays, prescription drugs, and some digital health tools, either partially or in full depending on the type of policy.

It is important to remember that **medications** include prescription drugs, over-the-counter drugs, and dietary supplements. Medications are designed to treat an illness, lessen a symptom, or prevent a disease. **Prescription drugs** require a written notice from a doctor, or prescription, before a pharmacy can release the medication into your care. **Dietary supplements** are products that you take by mouth to improve or manage your health. Unlike prescription drugs, they are generally available **over-the-counter** at a grocery store, drugstore, and online, and can be purchased without a prescription. These supplements include vitamins, minerals, herbs, powders, and liquids.

In order to save time, you may be asked to complete forms electronically ahead of your visit. Typically, these digital forms are available in your patient portal and some will require an electronic signature. An **electronic signature** is the digital equivalent of your handwritten signature and indicates that you agree to or accept the terms of the electronic document. If you have trouble accessing or completing digital forms, many medical offices still offer the opportunity to complete paper forms during your visit.

Another example of the paperless environment is electronic prescriptions. An **electronic prescription** is a computer-based version of the paper prescription doctors used to write by hand. Doctors now send it straight to the pharmacy of your choice.

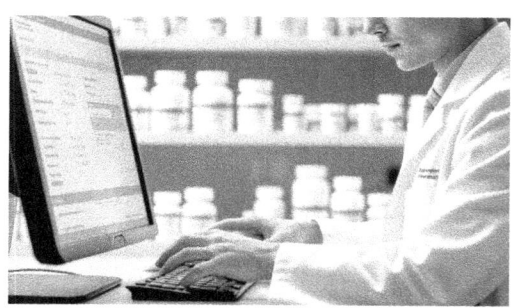
Electronic Prescription

There are many ways to get your medicine. The following chart highlights pharmacy options, support, and tools.

Pharmacy Type	How to Get Medicine	Works with Insurance?	Virtual Support	Other Tools
Retail	Pick up in person	Check with your provider	✗ Not usually	Basic reminders sent via text, smart pill boxes
Online	Delivered to your home	Check with your provider	✓ Often available by phone/video	Reminders, tracking apps, smart pill boxes
Mail-Order	Delivered by mail (often 90-day supply or more)	Check with your provider	✓ Some offer support	Some have tools and reminders

Before choosing a pharmacy, call your insurance company or check their website to see which ones are in-network. **In-network** means that your health insurance works with the pharmacy and will help pay for your prescription. If you go to an in-network pharmacy, it usually costs you less money than going to one that's not in your network.

Why bother with a paperless environment?
- Improved access to care, especially if you live in a rural environment
- Reduced costs
- Increased convenience
- Helps medical staff be more productive

What is driving this rapid shift?
- The move to virtual care, particularly during the COVID-19 pandemic
- Advances in **telehealth**

Telehealth is the use of technology to deliver care at a distance, or remotely. It is a broad term and includes all types of care given through technology — like video visits, phone calls, and apps. It helps doctors and patients share information and manage health online instead of with printed forms or in-person visits.

Telemedicine is part of telehealth. It refers to getting medical care from a doctor without going to the office, like through a video call.

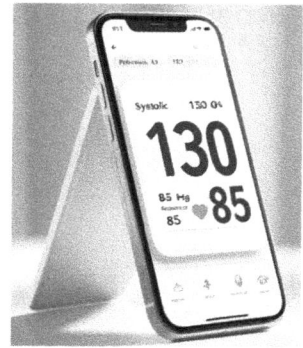
Mobile health apps are another part of telehealth. These are apps on your phone or tablet that help you track your health, collect information, or talk with healthcare providers. Some mobile health apps work with wearable devices. While the wearable device collects information like heart rate or steps, as discussed earlier, the app shows that data in a way that's easy to understand.

Howie's How-Tos on Preparing for Paperless Care

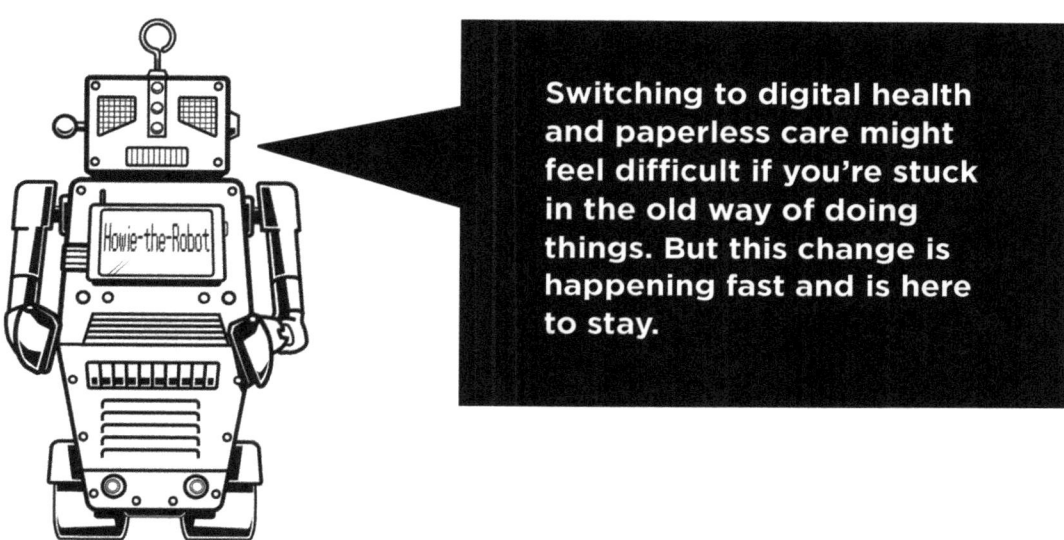

Switching to digital health and paperless care might feel difficult if you're stuck in the old way of doing things. But this change is happening fast and is here to stay.

Having the following resources will make the change easier for you.

1) An internet-connected device like a smartphone, tablet, laptop, or desktop computer.

2) Reliable, high-speed internet.

3) An email account.

4) A **username** and **strong password** that you can remember for accessing your patient portal.

5) Patience — unfortunately, digital health technologies do not always work the way we want them to when we need them; these technologies can have problems or stop working for a while.

Additionally, you should expect your providers to share this journey with you in a responsible way. A good provider of care will do the following:

- ✓ Provide clear instructions.
- ✓ Address your concerns.
- ✓ Communicate using plain language.
- ✓ Keep your health records safe and secure.
- ✓ Continue to provide paper-based forms, when requested, as you make the shift to paperless.

Activity #2

Directions: Read each question and provide the **best** answer.

1. Donald is about to have two extra teeth removed by his dentist. Before the procedure, his dentist asks which pharmacy to send a prescription for pain medicine. After his appointment, Donald plans to stop by his local grocery store to buy soft foods that are easy to chew. He likes how convenient the grocery store is and knows the pharmacy there has great service. Which pharmacy is Donald most likely to choose for his prescription?

    A) Amazon Pharmacy (online)
    B) Kroger Pharmacy (retail)
    C) Express Scripts (mail-order)

2. Alice likes that her insurance covers a 90-day supply of insulin and that it can be delivered to her home for free. Because her feet are often swollen and it's hard for her to get around, which pharmacy is she most likely to choose for her long-term medicine?

    A) Jackson's Neighborhood Pharmacy
    B) Express Scripts
    C) Kroger Pharmacy

3. Jack values having a face-to-face relationship with the medical professionals in his circle of care. He thinks it's best to get all his prescriptions from the same pharmacy chain. Today, Jack is leaving work early to pick up his arthritis medicine. Which pharmacy is he most likely going to after work?

    A) Jackson's Neighborhood Pharmacy
    B) Amazon Pharmacy
    C) Walgreens

4. Tabitha is reviewing a prescription bottle, which instructs her to take 1 tablet each day for 60 days. How many tablets will Tabitha take in 60 days?

    A) 30 tablets
    B) 60 tablets
    C) 120 tablets
    D) 240 tablets

5. What does it mean that Tabitha has 4 refills?

_____

_____

6. How can Tabitha use her patient portal to manage her prescription?

_____

_____

7. What is one way Tabitha's pharmacy might use technology to help her remember to take her medicine?

_____

_____

8. Which of the following is not likely to be found in a person's electronic health record (EHR)?

    A) Date of birth
    B) Insurance policy number
    C) Unshared home remedies
    D) Lab results

9. Based on the information in the passage, explain telehealth in your own words.

_____

_____

Activity #3

Directions: Peter, Maria, Jorge, Ivan, and Cathy want a mobile app to manage their health. Review each app below. Then, use the comments made by each individual to select the mobile health app that will help them achieve their goals.

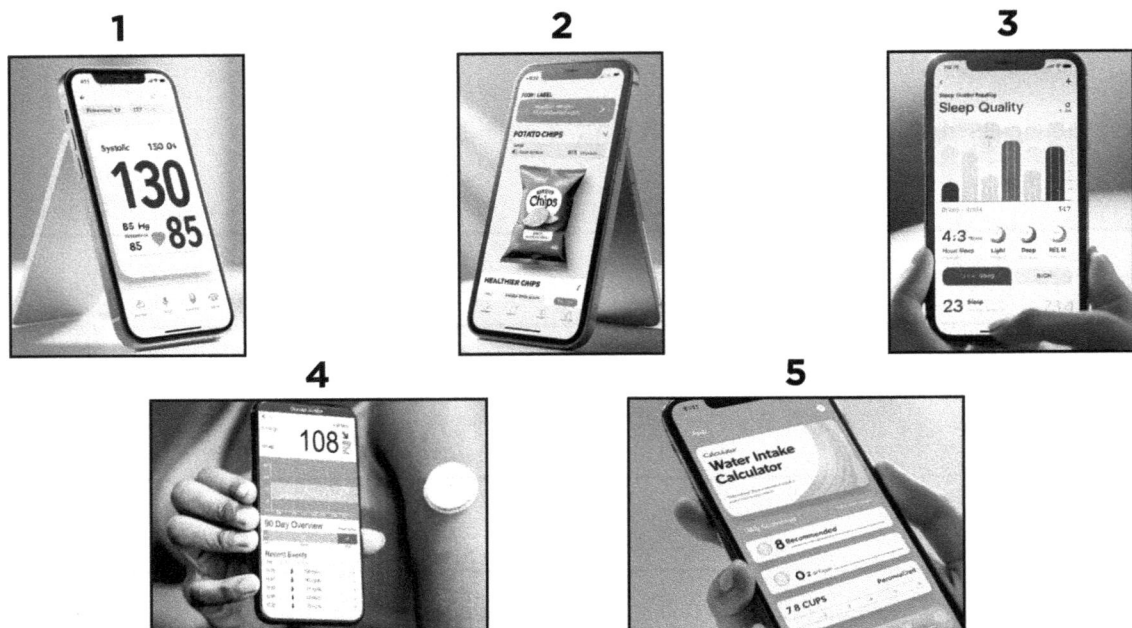

Patient	Comments	Best App (Write the Number)
Peter	"I need a way to see how my blood sugar changes during the day. I have type 2 diabetes and want to eat better to stay healthy."	
Maria	"My doctor told me I'm not drinking enough water. I need a reminder to help me drink the right amount each day based on my weight and daily activity."	
Jorge	"I want a tool that helps me take better care of my high blood pressure. I also want to learn what makes it go up or down."	
Ivan	"I don't sleep well. I want to track my sleep so I can learn how to improve my rest and make better choices."	
Cathy	"I love salty snacks! I'd like a tool I can use while shopping to scan foods and help me pick healthier options."	

Artificial Intelligence and Care

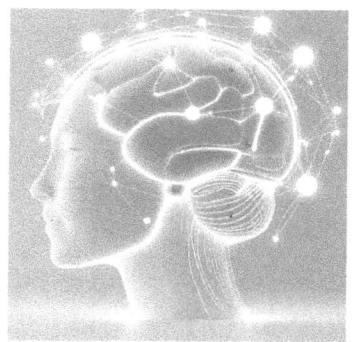

Artificial Intelligence, or AI, is a type of digital technology that helps machines do things that usually require human thinking. This includes learning, solving problems, understanding information, and making decisions. AI is the result of **data**. In healthcare, data includes important personal information like age, medical history, vital signs (such as heart rate and blood pressure), medications, allergies, lab tests, X-rays, and patient-reported information like symptoms, how treatments are working, and lifestyle habits. The following chart summarizes common symptoms and examples of lifestyle habits.

Symptoms	Lifestyle Habits
Cough	Healthy Diet
Tiredness	Physical Activity
Back Pain	Sleep
Vomiting	Regular Check-ups
Headache	Social Connections
Dizziness	Stress Management
Shortness of Breath	Tobacco Use
Skin Rash	Substance Abuse

As we live our lives, we create a lot of health information over time. AI is extremely good at looking through all that data, making sense of it, and using it to suggest helpful services and the best ways to deliver care.

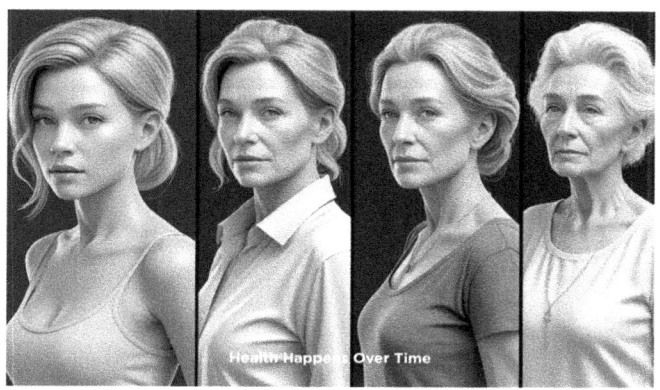

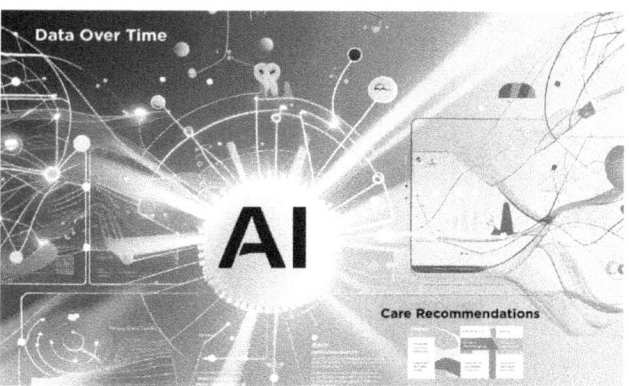

PAGE 21

Doctors can use the information from AI to decide whether to treat a patient and how to treat a patient.

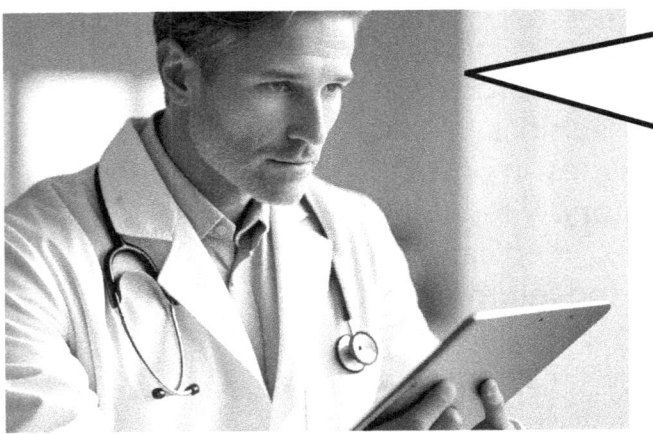

1. Does this patient need to be treated?
2. What treatment plan should I recommend?

Likewise, you now have these same tools to take care of your own health. You can learn about your health data like lab results and medications, take action to manage and improve your health, track your progress, and continue this process as you make choices to feel better. As the AI tool you're using learns more about you and your goals, it will get better at giving you helpful information made just for you. You can use this information to make better decisions and talk with your doctor about it.

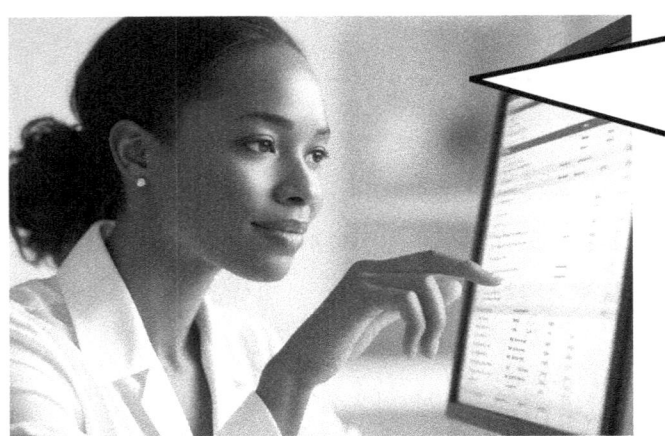

1. What information should I share and track?
2. Can I trust these tools to keep my data private?

Activity #4

Directions: Sofia is committed to making better health choices and is experimenting with AI to achieve this goal. You are invited to come along for the journey and learn with Sofia. Read each question and provide the **best** answer.

1. Sofia takes a picture of her dinner before eating the meal and shares a photo (in color) of the food on her plate with her favorite AI tool. She asks the AI to tell her about this meal.

   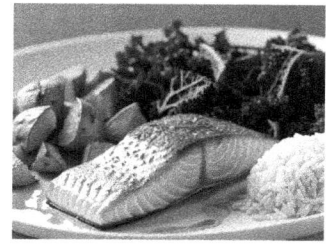

   True or **False**. Write **T** for True or **F** for False next to the statements below.

   _____ A) The AI tool is able to review the picture and identify every food on the plate.

   _____ B) When prompted, the AI is able to estimate the total calories of the entire meal.

2. Sofia's AI tool provides an overall meal assessment. Which of the following is not part of the meal assessment?

   A) Heart-healthy
   B) Diabetes-friendly (with portion control)
   C) Unbalanced
   D) Great for recovery

3. Which one of Sofia's food items is most likely described as being "good for heart and brain health?"

   A) Roasted Sweet Potatoes
   B) Grilled Salmon
   C) Steamed Kale

4. The AI tool identifies the following health benefits for one of Sofia's dinner items: good for eye health, digestion, and provides long-lasting energy. Which dinner item is most likely to have these benefits?

   A) Roasted Sweet Potatoes
   B) Grilled Salmon
   C) Steamed Kale

5. Based on the information that Sofia is receiving about her dinner from AI, how could you adopt this practice to make better decisions about what you eat over time?

___

Activity #5

Sofia desires to better understand a few of her lab results. She takes a picture with a smartphone of the test results and uploads them to her favorite AI tool.

Comp. Metabolic Panel (14)

Test	Current Result and Flag	Previous Result
Glucose[01]	86	78*
BUN[01]	12	14
Creatinine[01]	0.60	0.65

She asks the AI to provide feedback on her test results. Below is the response to her input data (i.e., photo and question), or **AI prompt**.

"These lab results come from a Comprehensive Metabolic Panel (CMP), which checks important markers of your overall health, especially kidney function, blood sugar, and hydration. Here's a quick summary of what your results mean." — ChatGPT

Glucose
o **Current:** 86   o **Previous:** 78 (marked with an asterisk, likely slightly low)   o **Normal range:** Usually about 70–99 mg/dL (fasting)   ✓ Your current level (86) is normal. It went up a bit from the last test, but that's okay — it's now in the healthy range.
BUN (Blood Urea Nitrogen)
o **Current:** 12   o **Previous:** 14   o **Normal range:** About 7–20 mg/dL   ✓ Your BUN level is normal and even improved slightly. This test checks how well your kidneys are working and if you're hydrated.
Creatinine
o **Current:** 0.60   o **Previous:** 0.65   o **Normal range:** About 0.6–1.2 mg/dL for adults   ✓ Still in the normal range. This is another marker of kidney health.

Directions: Read each question. Use the summary lab results above to provide the **best** answer.

1. Which test checks whether Sofia is getting enough **hydration**, or water?
    A) Glucose
    B) BUN
    C) Creatinine

2. Which test measures the amount of a simple sugar in the blood?
    A) Glucose
    B) BUN
    C) Creatinine

3. **True** or **False.** Write **T** for True or **F** for False next to the statements below.

    _____ A) Sofia's lab results communicate a positive update.

    _____ B) If Sofia has concerns about the accuracy of her summary results, she can ask the AI to share its sources.

4. What is an effective prompt, or question, Sofia can ask to learn how her diet may affect these lab results?

    _____

    _____

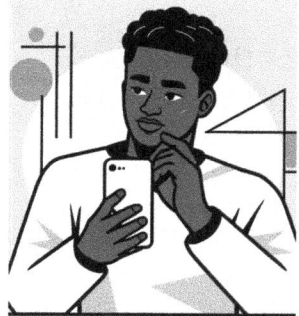

Show What You Know!

Congratulations on completing the lesson. You've made great progress. Enter your site code and the information below to answer a few quick questions about what you learned.

| Lesson One | Checkpoint Number: **2** |

Key Terms

AI Prompt	Input data, which can include instructions, a question, images, code, video, and other information needed to get a response.
Artificial Intelligence	A type of digital technology that helps machines do things that usually require human thinking.
Chatbot	A virtual assistant that uses artificial intelligence to answer questions, access healthcare information, and connect an individual with the right medical professional.
Circle of Care	A support system that connects you with people, places, meaningful technology, and your health information.
Data	Information related to your health, medical history, and care experiences.
Dietary Supplement	A product that you take by mouth to improve or manage your health.
Digital Health	Using technology like phones, computers, or apps to take care of your health, talk to a doctor, get medicine, and learn how to stay healthy.
Electronic Health Record (EHR)	A digital version of a patient's medical history.
Electronic Prescription	A computer-based version of the paper prescription that doctors send straight to a pharmacy.
Electronic Signature	The digital equivalent of a handwritten signature.
E-Visit	A way to safely give and receive information about your health virtually, without interacting with an individual directly.

Health Insurance	A type of coverage that pays your medical bills when you get sick or injured.
Hydration	A condition where the body has enough water to function properly.
In-Network	The health insurance coverage works with the care provider and will help pay for medical costs.
Medicaid	Insurance coverage for low-income individuals and families.
Medicare	A federal health insurance program for people 65 years of age and older.
Medication	A prescription drug, over-the-counter drug, or dietary supplement.
Mobile Health App	A software program used on a smartphone or tablet that helps you track your health, collect information, or talk with healthcare providers.
Over-the-Counter	Available for purchase without a prescription.
Patient Portal	A secure website or app that lets users review their health information.
Prescription Drug	A substance that requires a written notice from a doctor before a pharmacy can release the medication into the individual's care.
Telehealth	The use of technology to deliver care remotely.
Telemedicine	Medical care from a doctor without an in-person visit.
Video Call	A live virtual visit with a doctor.
Virtual Reality	A computer-made world that you can explore and interact with.
Wearable Device	An electronic gadget connected to the internet and worn on the body.

LESSON TWO: Online Patient Portals

Introduction

Objectives – After completing this lesson, you will be able to:
- Start using your patient portal
- Access online health information when you can't remember your password
- Explain how to share health records in your patient portal
- Figure out where to go to do things like send messages, see test results, or manage appointments
- Identify common health screenings recommended for older adults

Key Terms

- Cervix
- Colonoscopy
- Colorectal Cancer
- Main Dashboard
- Mammogram
- Osteoporosis
- Patient Portal
- Peer-Reviewed Study
- Preventive Care
- Prostate
- Provider
- Proxy Access
- Rectum

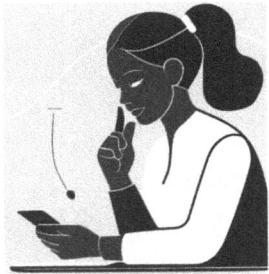

Let's Get Started!

Your voice matters. Enter your site code and the information below to share what you already know and what you hope to learn about online patient portals.

| Lesson Two | Checkpoint Number: **3** |

Getting Started

As discussed in the previous lesson, a **patient portal** is a secure website that provides access to your health information. In order to start using a patient portal, you need a link to your care provider's patient portal, a smartphone, tablet, or computer, and an email address and strong password to create an account.

Surveys and **peer-reviewed studies**, which is research checked by experts before publication, show that many people have concerns about using a patient portal.[1] They may wonder if it will be useful, if their information will stay private and safe, or if they have the internet and devices they need to use it. The questions and answers below can help you get started and know what to expect.

Frequently Asked Questions (FAQs)

1) How do I access the patient portal?

Answer: You can get to the patient portal by going to the website your doctor's office gives you. Some places also have an app you can download to your phone or tablet.

2) How do I log in?

Answer: You will need a username and password. If you don't have one yet, you will need to set up an account using a username and password that you can remember or easily access when needed.

3) What can I do inside the portal?

Answer: You can see test results, send messages to your doctor, ask for medicine refills, review billing statements and payments, and schedule appointments.

4) Is the patient portal safe to use?

Answer: Yes. Typically, the portal is protected with passwords and other safety tools to help keep your health information private.

The R.E.E.L.

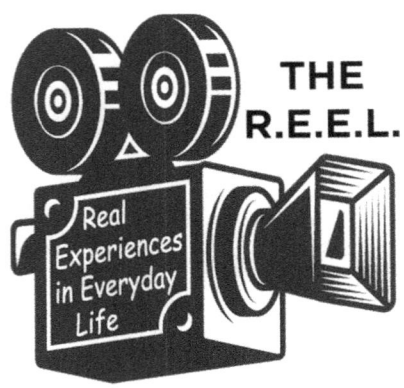

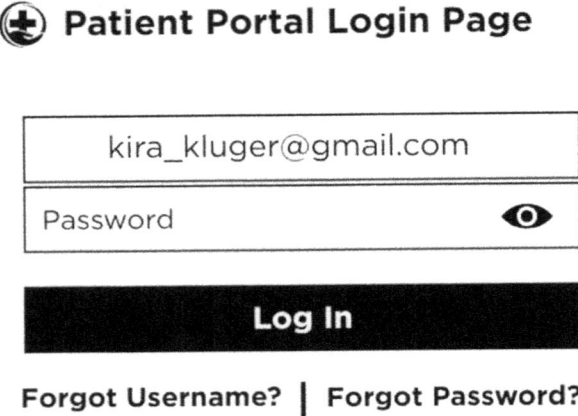

Directions: Kira wants to log in to her patient portal. She remembers her username, but can't remember her password. What should she do? Use the Patient Portal Login Page image to assist you.

_____

_____

Activity #1

Directions: Figure 2-1 presents a sample login page for a patient portal. Review the information and provide the **best** answer for the questions that follow.

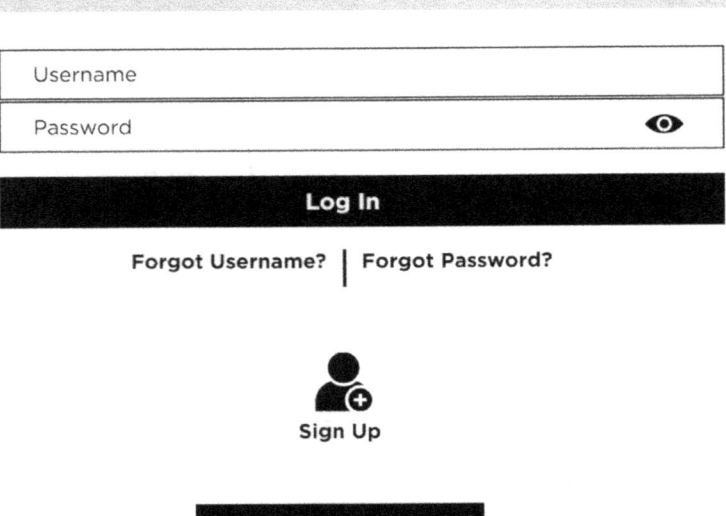

Figure 2-1: Sample Patient Portal Login Page

1. Which of the following helps the system supporting the patient portal know who you are?

    A) Insurance policy number

    B) Date of birth

    C) Username

    D) Password

2. Why would a user click on the "eye" icon when logging in to the portal?

    A) To reset their password

    B) To see the password they are typing

    C) To check the number of characters in their password

    D) To see how strong their password is

3. Kameron wants online access to his health records. He has never used his patient portal before. What should he do to get started?

    A) Type his email address in the username field

    B) Log in

    C) Click the "Forgot Username" link

    D) Sign up

4. Sandra can't remember her password and clicks on the "Forgot Password" link. What is most likely to happen next?

    A) She will be asked to call a support number for help.

    B) She will be asked to check her email to reset her password.

    C) She will be asked to create a new account.

    D) None of the above

5. Why would a user choose the "pay as guest" option?

    A) They don't have an account yet, but need to pay a bill quickly.

    B) They only need to make a one-time payment and don't plan to use the portal often.

    C) They are helping a family member pay a bill.

    D) All of the above

Inside the Portal

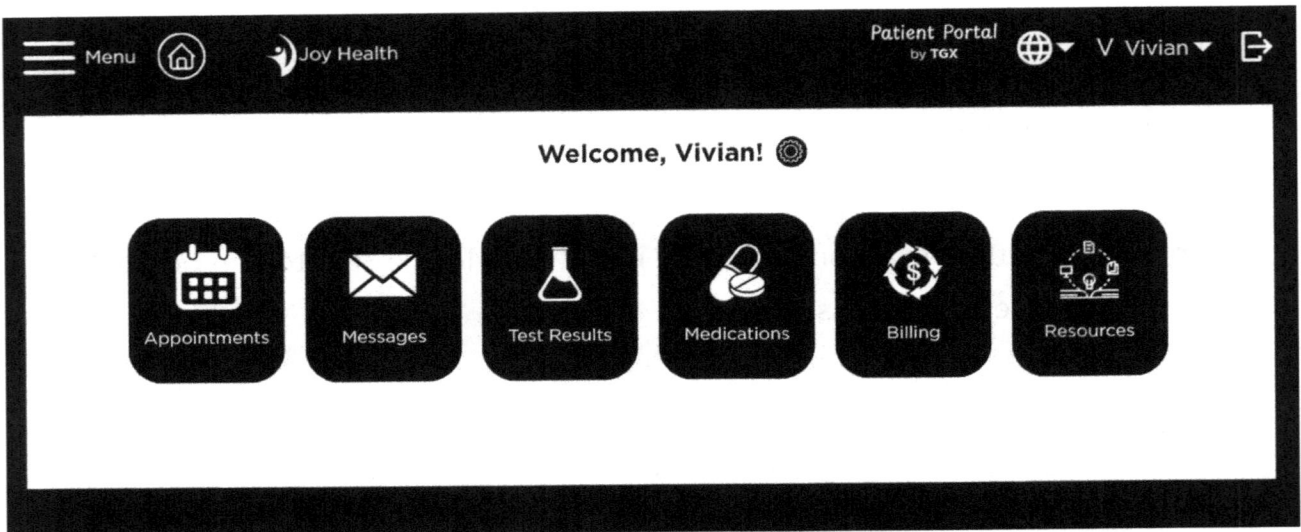

Figure 2-2: Sample Patient Portal

You have logged in to your patient portal. What do you do next? Patient portals are designed to help you stay involved in your care and get answers in a secure environment without needing to call or visit the doctor's office. Your doctor may send you an email and direct you to your patient portal to read a private message about your health. You might want to see the date and time of your next appointment. As mentioned earlier, you may simply need to look at what you owe and pay a bill quickly.

The chart below explains some of the features shown in **Figure 2-2**.

Click and Know: What Your Patient Portal Will Show	
Appointments	Check when and where your next visit is.
Billing Summary	Look at what you owe and pay bills online.
Care Team	Locate names, roles, and contact information for your providers.
Friends and Family Access	Review the people who have permission to view your records and help with care.

Click and Know: What Your Patient Portal Will Show	
Medical History	Review past visits, diagnoses, or surgeries.
Medications	View what medicines you're taking and when to take them.
Messages	Read replies or updates from your care team.
Preventive Care	Find your next due date for a screening test like a colonoscopy or mammogram.
Shot Records	See what vaccines you've had and if you're due for any.
Test Results	See your lab work or X-ray results.

Preventive care represents the steps you take to stay healthy and find problems early. These steps include regular check-ups, shots, and screening tests that help catch diseases before you feel sick. The two screening tests mentioned in the table are colonoscopy and mammogram. A **colonoscopy** is a type of test where a doctor looks inside the large intestine (colon) using a thin, flexible tube with a camera to check for problems like cancer or polyps. A **mammogram** is another preventive care measure where an X-ray picture of the breast is taken to find signs of breast cancer early.

Once you start exploring your patient portal, you will also discover education resources. You might find articles, short videos, or tips for staying healthy. Some portals even give advice on eating better, managing stress, or dealing with chronic illnesses like diabetes. These tools can help you feel more informed and confident about your care.

The features provided in your patient portal will vary according to decisions made by your doctor or healthcare organization. Providers choose tools based on what their patients need. They also decide whether to turn an option on or off. Thus, it's important to tell your provider what you want your patient portal to do for you. In a care setting, a **provider** is a licensed professional like a doctor, dentist, nurse, pharmacist, or therapist. It also includes places that deliver care such as a hospital, clinic, nursing home, or laboratory.

Make sure to share your thoughts with your doctor and fill out surveys so they know what you think and need.

Howie's How-Tos on Friends and Family Access

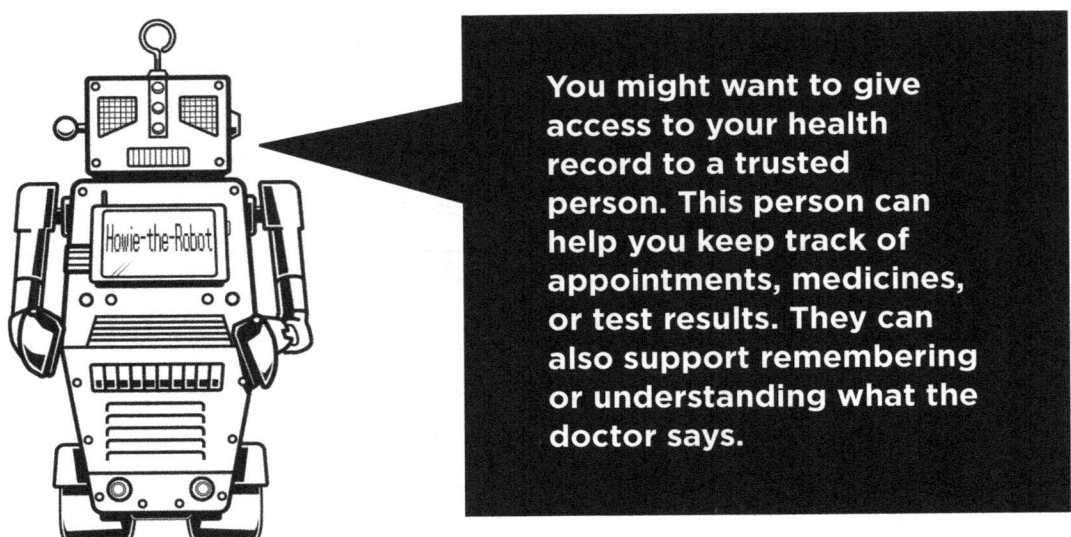

You might want to give access to your health record to a trusted person. This person can help you keep track of appointments, medicines, or test results. They can also support remembering or understanding what the doctor says.

Below are simple steps you can follow to give a trusted person access to your health record through your patient portal.

1) Log in to your patient portal.
2) Find the "Sharing" or "Friends and Family Access" section.
3) Click "Add a person" or "Give access."
4) Enter the person's name and email address.
5) Choose the parts of your health record you want them to see.
6) Save and confirm your choice.

If you no longer wish to grant access to this person, you can remove that person from your patient portal. Return to the "Sharing" or "Friends and Family Access" section or Settings menu. Look for an option that mentions shared access, proxy access, or manage permissions to update their access status. **Proxy access** means giving another person like a family member or caregiver permission to see and help you manage your health information online.

Activity #2

Directions: Look closely at **Figure 2-3**. The numbers in the picture point to different parts of the patient portal and what they do. Read each question carefully and circle the answer that best matches what you see in the picture and what you've learned about using a patient portal.

Figure 2-3: Patient Portal Diagram

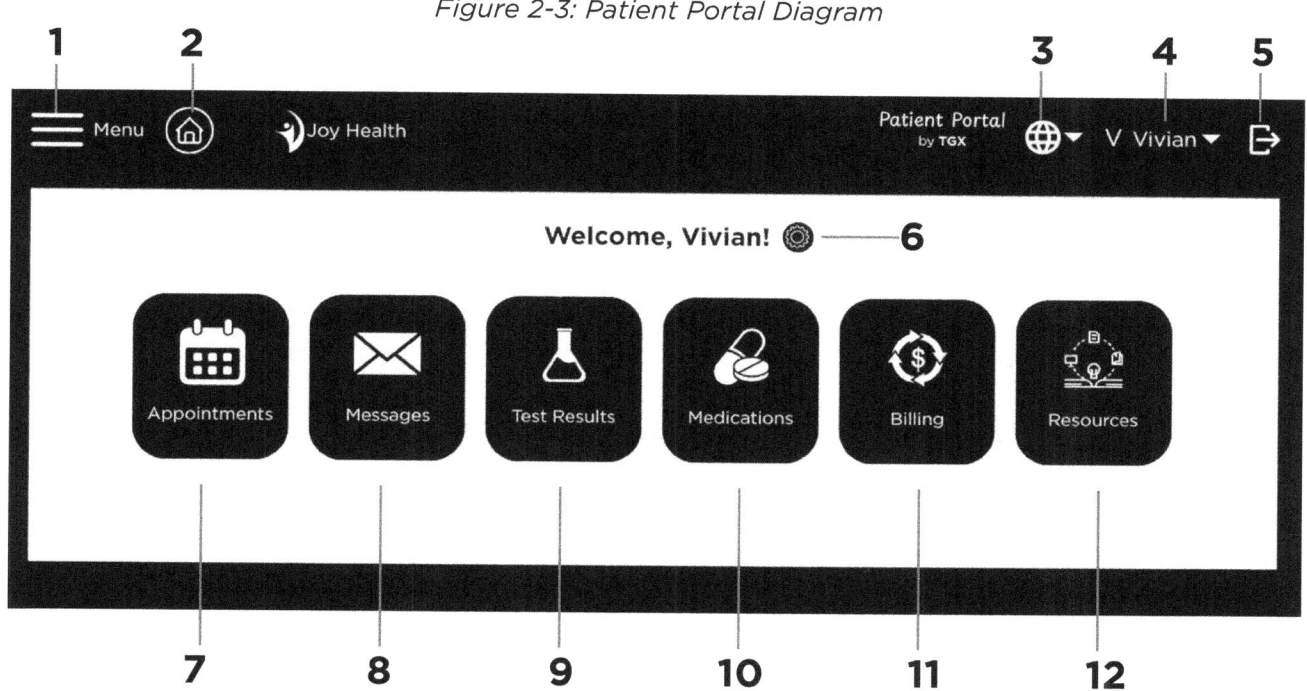

1. Which labels shows where to find the date of your next doctor's visit?

    A) Label 2   B) Label 3   C) Label 7

2. Where can you check if you have a bill from your last doctor's visit?

    A) Label 1   B) Label 11   C) Label 12

3. Which label shows where to change your password?

    A) Label 2   B) Label 4   C) Labels 4 and 6

4. Which label shows where to click to log out of the patient portal?

    A) Label 1   B) Label 5   C) Label 6

5. Where can you find a full list of menu options?
   A) Label 1   B) Label 6   C) Label 12

6. Which label lets you change the language to Spanish?
   A) Label 3   B) Label 4   C) Label 6

7. Which label shows the trends from your last 5 lab tests?
   A) Label 4   B) Label 8   C) Label 9

8. Where do you go to send a private message about your health to your doctor?
   A) Label 1   B) Label 4   C) Label 8

9. Which label allows you to view your main dashboard? *Note:* The **main dashboard** presents important information in one place and is the first page you see after you log in.
   A) Label 1   B) Label 2   C) Labels 5

10. Which label takes you to your list of prescriptions or medicines?
    A) Label 4   B) Label 9   C) Label 10

11. Where do you go to let a trusted family member or caregiver see your health information in the patient portal?
    A) Label 4   B) Label 8   C) Label 12

12. Which label takes you to videos and articles your doctor thinks will help you stay healthy?
    A) Label 3   B) Label 8   C) Label 12

Activity #3

Preventive Screenings

Directions: In this lesson, you learned how patient portals can help you stay on track with preventive care. The activity below shows common health screenings for older adults. Draw a line to match each screening with the reason it helps individuals stay healthy. Use the tips on the following page to assist you.

Screening	Reason
Blood Pressure	Checks for signs of blood sugar levels being too high.
Cholesterol	Finds early signs of colon cancer when it's easiest to treat.
Diabetes	Measures fat in your blood that can raise the risk of heart attack or stroke.
Colorectal Cancer	Detects hearing loss that can affect safety, memory, and communication.
Mammogram	Checks bone strength to help prevent serious breaks or fractures.
Osteoporosis	Checks for low levels that can weaken bones and raise the risk of falls or breaks.
Vitamin D	Looks for early signs of breast cancer before you feel a lump.
Prostate Exam	Screens for depression or memory loss to support brain and emotional health.
Vision	Checks for when the heart is working too hard to push blood, which can lead to heart problems or a stroke.
Pap Smear	Helps find eye problems that can lead to vision loss or falls.
Hearing	Checks for cancerous cells in the cervix.
Mental Health	Looks for signs of problems in a small gland in men that helps make fluid for reproduction.

Tips:

- The **cervix** is part of the female reproductive system that connects the uterus, or womb, to the birth canal.
- **Colorectal cancer** is a type of cancer that starts in the last part of the large intestine, or **rectum**, where poop is stored before it leaves the body.
- The **prostate** is a small gland in men that is similar to the size of a walnut and sits just below the bladder. As men get older, the prostate can grow larger, which sometimes causes problems with urination.
- **Osteoporosis** is a condition where bones become thin and weak, making them more likely to break.

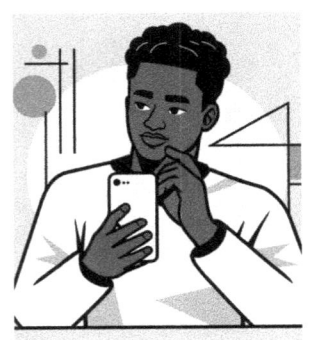

Show What You Know!

Congratulations on completing the lesson. You've made great progress. Enter your site code and the information below to answer a few quick questions about what you learned.

| Lesson Two | Checkpoint Number: **4** |

Key Terms

Cervix	Part of the female reproductive system that connects the uterus, or womb, to the birth canal.
Colonoscopy	A type of test where a doctor looks inside the large intestine (colon) using a thin, flexible tube with a camera to check for problems like cancer or polyps.
Colorectal Cancer	A type of cancer that starts in the last part of the large intestine where poop is stored before it leaves the body.
Main Dashboard	The central location in your patient portal that allows you to access your health information.
Mammogram	A preventive care measure where an X-ray picture of the breast is taken to find signs of breast cancer early.
Osteoporosis	A condition where bones become thin and weak, making them more likely to break.
Patient Portal	A secure website that provides access to health information.
Peer-Reviewed Study	A research report that other experts check before it gets published.
Preventive Care	Actions taken to stay healthy and find problems early before feeling sick or developing symptoms.
Prostate	A small, walnut-shaped gland in men that sits just below the bladder.
Provider	A doctor, nurse, clinic, or hospital that gives medical care.
Proxy Access	Giving another person like a family member or caregiver permission to see and help you manage your health information online.
Rectum	The last part of the large intestine where poop is stored before it leaves the body.

LESSON THREE: Telehealth Visits

Introduction

Objectives – After completing this lesson, you will be able to:
- Book an appointment with your doctor online
- Describe protected health information, or PHI
- Explain how to use generative AI to help you prepare for a telehealth visit
- Practice asking AI for help to prepare good questions for your doctor
- Fix common technical problems that can occur during a telehealth visit

Key Terms

- Diabetes
- Generative AI
- HIPAA
- Hypertension
- Protected Health Information
- Tech-for-Care Advocate
- Telehealth
- Telehealth Visit

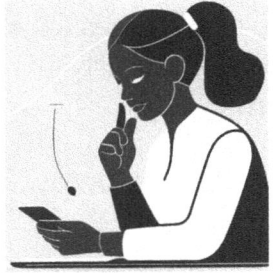

Let's Get Started!

Your voice matters. Enter your site code and the information below to share what you already know and what you hope to learn about telehealth visits.

| Lesson Three | Checkpoint Number: **5** |

Online Scheduling

In Lesson One we defined **telehealth** as the use of technology to deliver care at a distance, or remotely. Online scheduling allows patients to book an appointment at their convenience. Many doctor websites have a menu, button, or link you can click to make an appointment. Once you click the link, you will choose a doctor and answer a few questions to find the best times.

Step 1: Book an Appointment

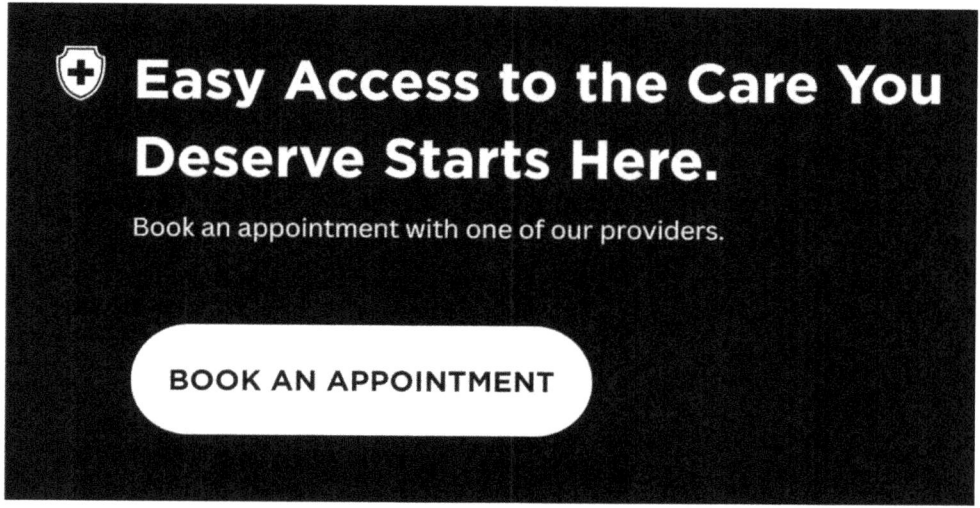

Step 2: Select a Provider

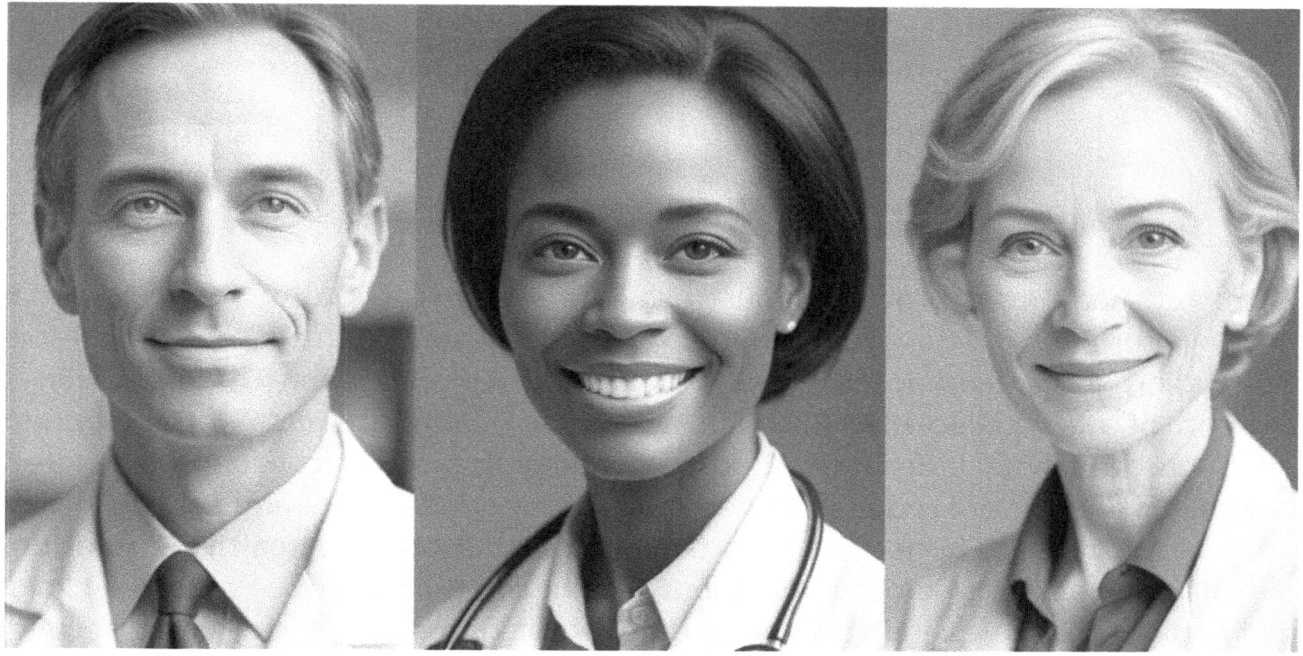

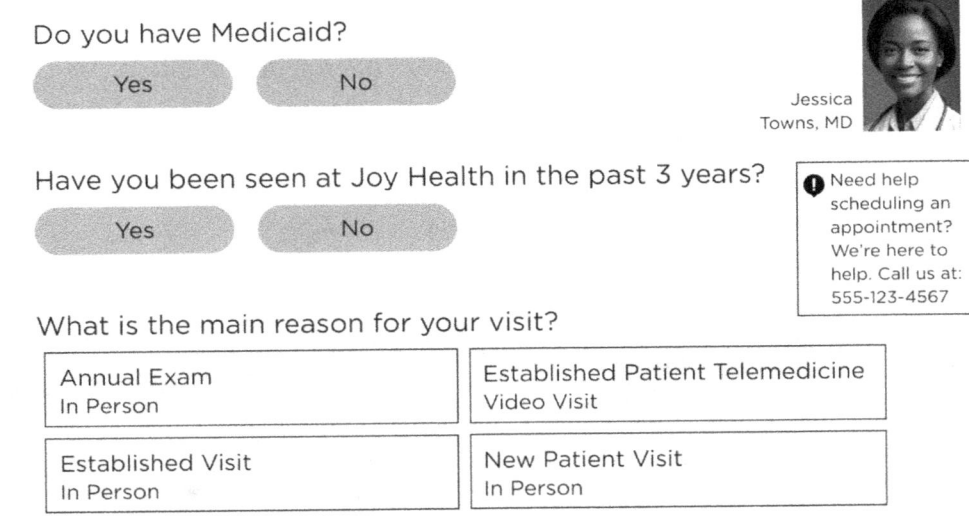

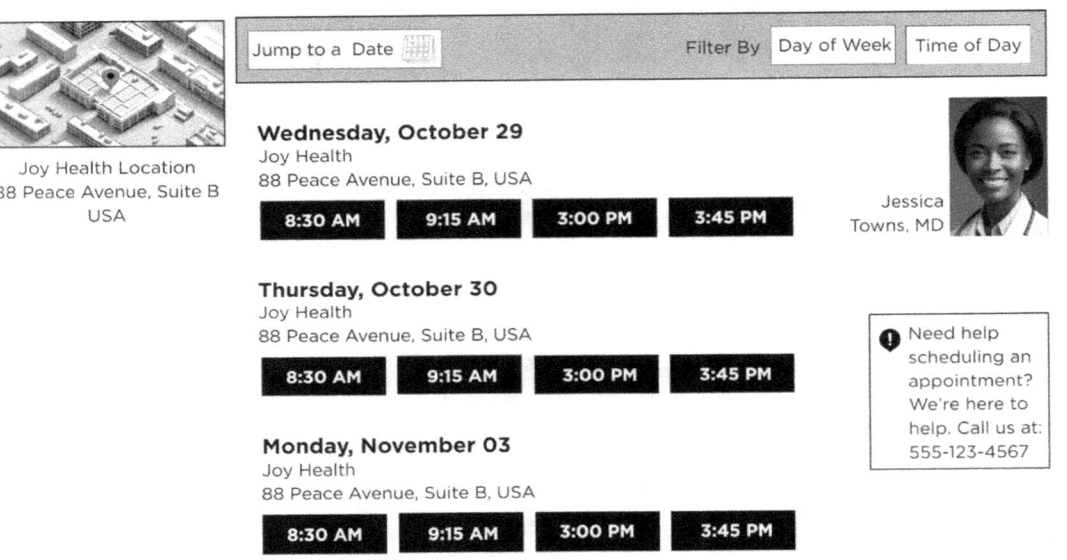

Trusted healthcare providers must use safe systems to protect your personal health information when you schedule online. These systems use strong tools like coding and locked access to keep your information private. These guidelines are part of a law called **HIPAA**, which stands for Health Insurance Portability and Accountability Act. Under HIPAA, online scheduling systems collecting protected health information are required to keep this information private and secure. If they do not, they can face huge fines or be taken to court. **Protected health information,** or PHI, is any personal information about your health that is kept by a doctor, clinic, or hospital. Examples include name, date of birth, medical history, test results, medications, and appointments.

Activity #1

Directions: Read each question and provide the **best** answer.

1. Which of the following is a benefit of booking a doctor's appointment online?

    A) You have to wait on hold to talk to someone.

    B) You can see available options and choose a time that works best for you.

    C) You must email staff to confirm the doctor's availability.

    D) You need to list all your symptoms before scheduling an appointment.

2. How is a doctor's visit for an *established patient* likely different from a *new patient*?

    A) A new patient pays less for their first visit.

    B) A new patient gets to go to the front of the line with no waiting.

    C) An established patient may not need to fill out as many forms.

    D) An established patient always sees a different doctor.

3. Why is it necessary to select a provider before choosing a date and time?

    A) So the system knows your favorite doctor.

    B) So you can see how long the visit will take.

    C) So the doctor can match their schedule with your availability.

    D) So the system can match you with the doctor's available times.

4. During the online scheduling process, why is the patient asked if they have seen their provider in the last 3 years?

    A) To know if the patient remembers their last visit.

    B) To decide if the patient is new or returning.

    C) To find out if the patient has moved.

    D) To see if the patience has updated insurance information.

5. **True** or **False**. Write **T** for True or **F** for False next to the statements below.

    _____ a) When scheduling an appointment online, you can jump to a future month.

_____ b) When booking an appointment online, you will need to enter personal details like your name, date of birth, and contact information.

_____ c) Patients who schedule a doctor's appointment online are more likely to miss their visit.

_____ d) You can use online scheduling anytime — day or night.

_____ e) Karen reports taking vitamin B12 on a regular basis and this information is included in her electronic health record. Karen's use of vitamin B12 tablets is not considered protected health information.

PREPARING FOR YOUR VISIT

Now that you know how to book an appointment online, it is important to prepare for your telehealth visit. A **telehealth visit**, or video call, with your doctor can take place on your phone, tablet, or computer. Generally, you will talk about your health concerns, just like in a regular visit, and may get advice, prescriptions, or next steps. It is important to be in a quiet place with good internet and have any questions or health information ready.

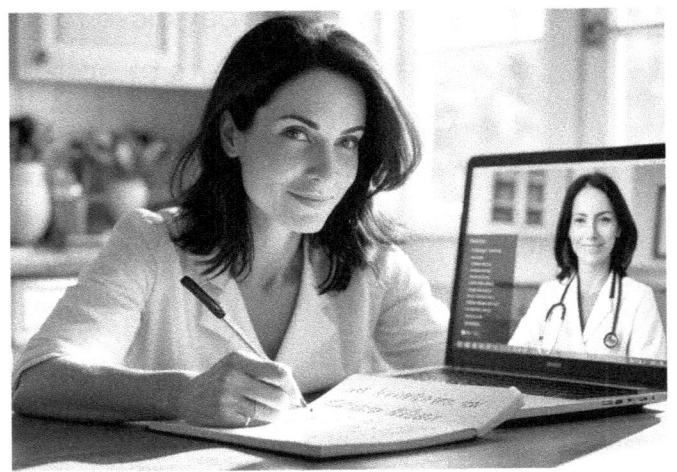

Using Generative AI

Sometimes talking to a doctor can feel scary, especially if you don't know the right medical words to explain your concerns. You are a significant part of your care team (remember **Lesson One** and the **Circle of Care**), and there are tools that can help make things easier. If it feels hard to think of questions to ask your doctor, use generative AI as your helper to gain practice and build confidence. **Generative AI** is a type of computer program that can create text, images, audio, voice, videos, or code. As explained in Lesson One, once you give it a question or idea, it will generate, or make, a response based on what it has learned.

The following table highlights AI prompts that you can use to organize your thoughts. As a review, an AI prompt is a question or instructions you type to ask a computer program (like ChatGPT, Claude, or Gemini) for help or information. It's like starting a conversation with the computer so it knows how to respond.

Get Ready for Your Telehealth Visit: Easy AI Prompts to Help You Prepare
1) I'm feeling tired and dizzy — how can I describe this clearly?
2) What should I ask during a check-up for high blood pressure?
3) Please help me list questions to ask my doctor about my lower back pain.
4) How can I describe my sleep problems in a clear way?
5) Help me describe my emotional health to my doctor, including how often I feel sad, tired, or anxious, and how it's affecting my appetite and daily life.
6) How can I keep track of times when I've had trouble thinking clearly, remembering things, or staying focused so I can share them with my doctor?
7) During my sister's last visit, her doctor summarized her condition as chronic fatigue syndrome. Can you explain this to me in plain language?

It is important to exercise caution when using AI to help you with your health. Applications like ChatGPT can help you think through your health questions, but they aren't private like your doctor's office. Also, as a general-purpose tool, they are not under HIPAA. So, use them with caution and do not type in your full name, birthdate, or any other personal information that could identify you. Use general terms like "my friend" or "someone I know," keeping it simple. Finally, always talk to your doctor before making decisions about your health.

The R.E.E.L.

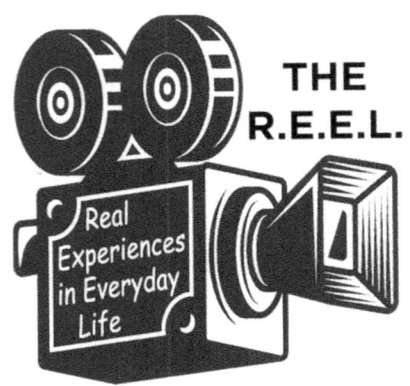

Tech-for-Care Advocate

Melissa is a tech-for-care advocate, or TCA, assisting Nate, who is 25 years old. Nate recently checked his patient portal and found a message from his doctor. The doctor is concerned about his high blood pressure (**hypertension**), high blood sugar (**diabetes**), and a lab result showing his creatinine is higher than normal. Nate has a telehealth appointment scheduled to go over his lab results, but he feels nervous and unsure about what to do with this information and how to engage with his doctor.

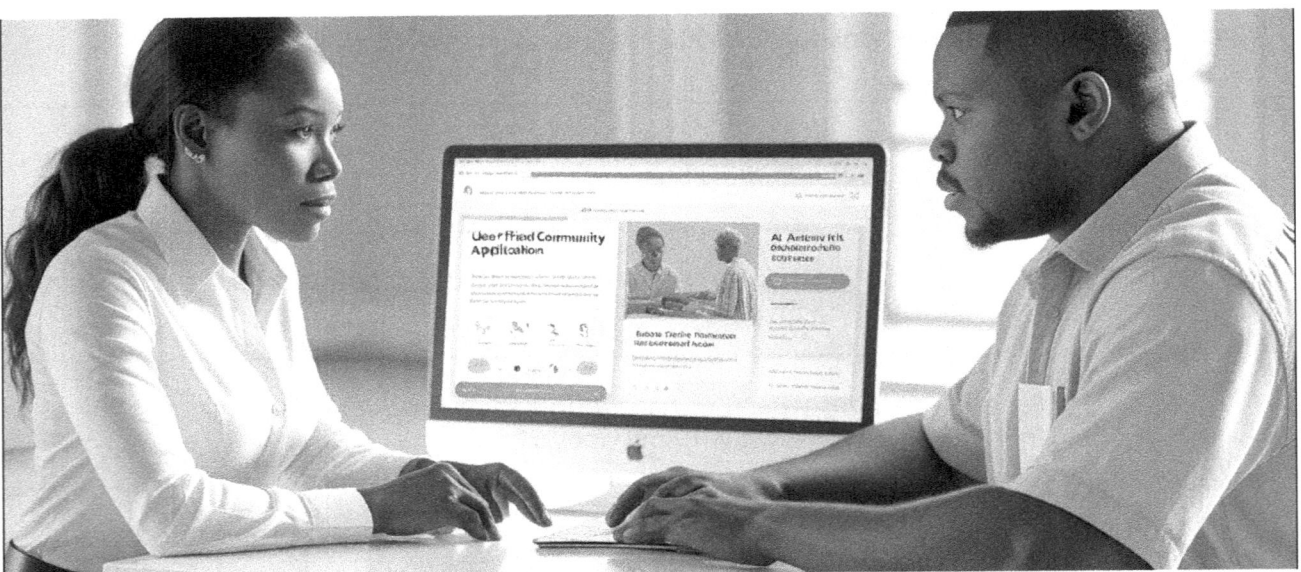

Note: A **tech-for-care advocate** is someone who helps people use technology to manage their health and speak up for their care needs.

Directions: Melissa wants to show Nate how to use AI to organize his thoughts and understand his health better. What AI prompts can Melissa and Nate develop together that will help him feel ready to talk about his care with his doctor?

_____

_____

Checking In

On the day of your telehealth visit, it is important to check in 15 minutes early and have all of your important information handy, including questions you plan on asking. Your doctor might send you a link to the video meeting. In some instances, you may be able to click a link at your doctor's website to check in for your call.

Telemedicine Links

When you log in or check in, test your device camera and microphone to ensure that they work. Generally, the video and microphone images appearing on the screen will indicate whether these features are on or off, or working or not working.

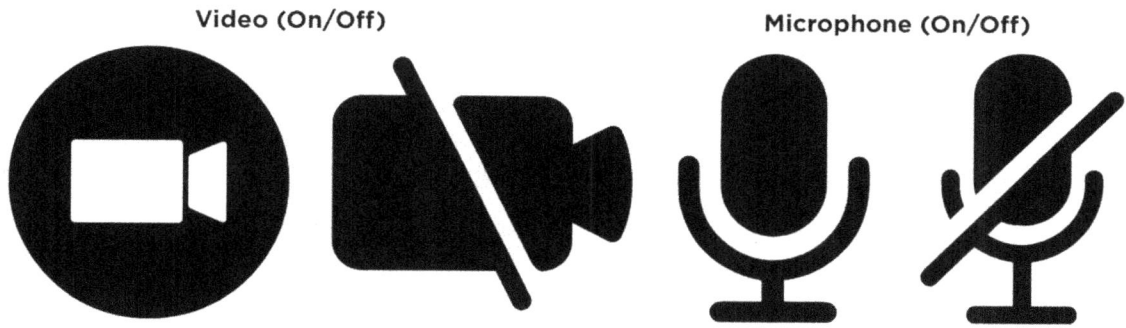

If you experience difficulty, check your camera and video settings, make sure you have access to the internet, and restart the application if problems continue.

Activity #2

Directions: Read each question and provide the **best** answer.

1. **Fill in the Blank.** Before a telehealth visit it's a good idea to _____.

    A) organize your medicines.

    B) write down concerns about your health.

    C) turn off your phone to avoid distractions.

    D) jot down how many hours you slept the night before.

2. **Fill in the Blank.** Generative AI is similar to having a smart helper that can write, draw, or explain things in response to a _____ that you enter.

    A) question

    B) prompt

    C) idea

    D) problem

3. How might a doctor's office confirm your identity during a telehealth visit?

    A) They will ask you to show a photo ID on camera.

    B) They will ask for your date of birth.

    C) They will ask for your home address.

    D) All of the above.

4. Pam is preparing for a scheduled telehealth visit with her doctor. She needs your help figuring out the best course of action to take in order to get ready. Correctly order each step from one (1) to five (5) with one being the first step and five being the last step.

Step	Order (1 to 5)
Click the link to enter the virtual waiting room	
Test your device camera and microphone	
Check In	
Write down questions beforehand	
Find a quiet, private space	

Activity #3

Directions: Tom Jackson is about to check in for his telehealth visit. **Figure 3-1** presents a screenshot of the welcome screen used by Tom's doctor's office for telehealth check-ins. Review **Figure 3-1** and answer the questions that follow.

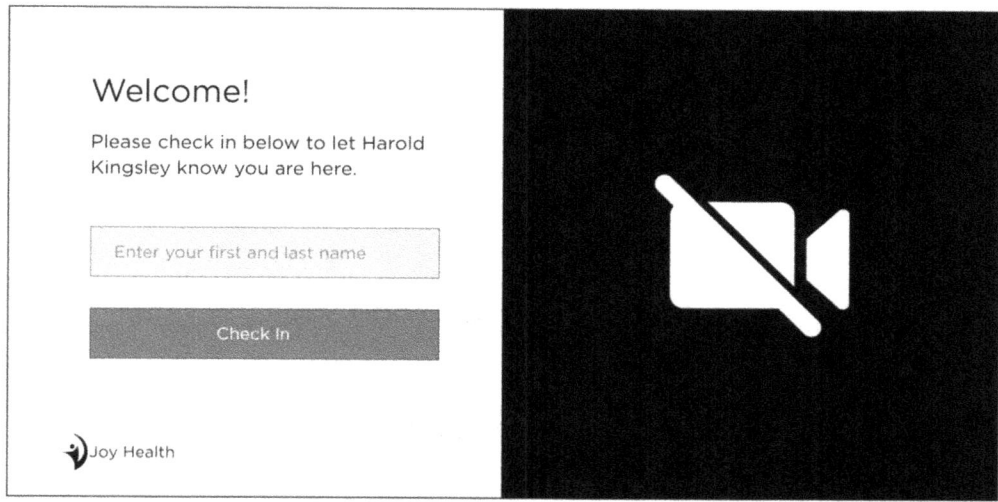

Figure 3-1: Joy Health Telehealth Check In

1. Which doctor is Tom visiting?

    A) Dr. Kingsley   B) Dr. Towns   C) Dr. Wyatt

2. What must Tom do in order to check in?

    A) Turn on his camera   B) Enter his last name   C) Enter "Tom Jackson"

3. When Tom's doctor appears, Tom can see and hear his doctor, but his doctor can't hear him. What is the best thing Tom can do to fix the problem?

    A) Click the link in the appointment reminder email

    B) Check his audio settings

    C) Switch to a different browser

4. Five minutes into the virtual visit, Tom's video freezes. What is the best thing Tom can do to fix the problem?

    A) Leave the visit and call his doctor's office

    B) Turn off his camera and hope it starts working again

    C) Check his internet connection and try to reconnect

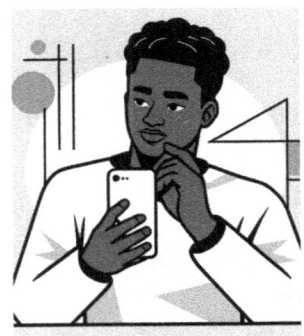

Show What You Know!

Congratulations on completing the lesson. You've made great progress. Enter your site code and the information below to answer a few quick questions about what you learned.

| Lesson Three | Checkpoint Number: **6** |

Key Terms

Diabetes — High blood sugar.

Generative AI — A type of computer program that can create text, images, audio, voice, videos, or code once prompted.

HIPAA — Refers to the Health Insurance Portability and Accountability Act, which requires providers to keep protected health information private and secure.

Hypertension — High blood pressure.

Protected Health Information — Any personal information about your health that is kept by a doctor, clinic, or hospital.

Tech-for-Care Advocate — Someone who helps people use technology to manage their health and speak up for their care needs.

Telehealth — The use of technology to deliver care at a distance, or remotely.

Telehealth Visit — A video call with your doctor that you can do instead of going to the office.

LESSON FOUR: Everyday Care

Introduction

Objectives – After completing this lesson, you will be able to:
- Explain types of mobile health apps
- Find safe and reliable health apps
- Identify the amount of sugar in popular beverages
- Describe common health signs tracked with remote patient monitoring
- Consider how your circle of care can support safe, independent living

Key Terms

- Aging In Place
- AI Chatbot
- Biosensor
- Continuous Glucose Monitor
- COPD
- Kombucha
- Mobile Health App

- Oxygen Saturation
- Patient-Reported Outcome
- Pulse Oximeter
- Remote Patient Monitoring
- Vital Signs
- Wearable

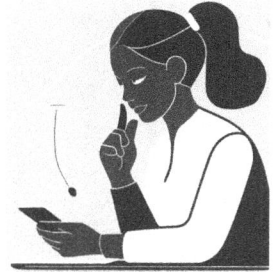

Let's Get Started!

Your voice matters. Enter your site code and the information below to share what you already know and what you hope to learn about health apps and remote patient monitoring.

| Lesson Four | Checkpoint Number: 7 |

Mobile Health Apps

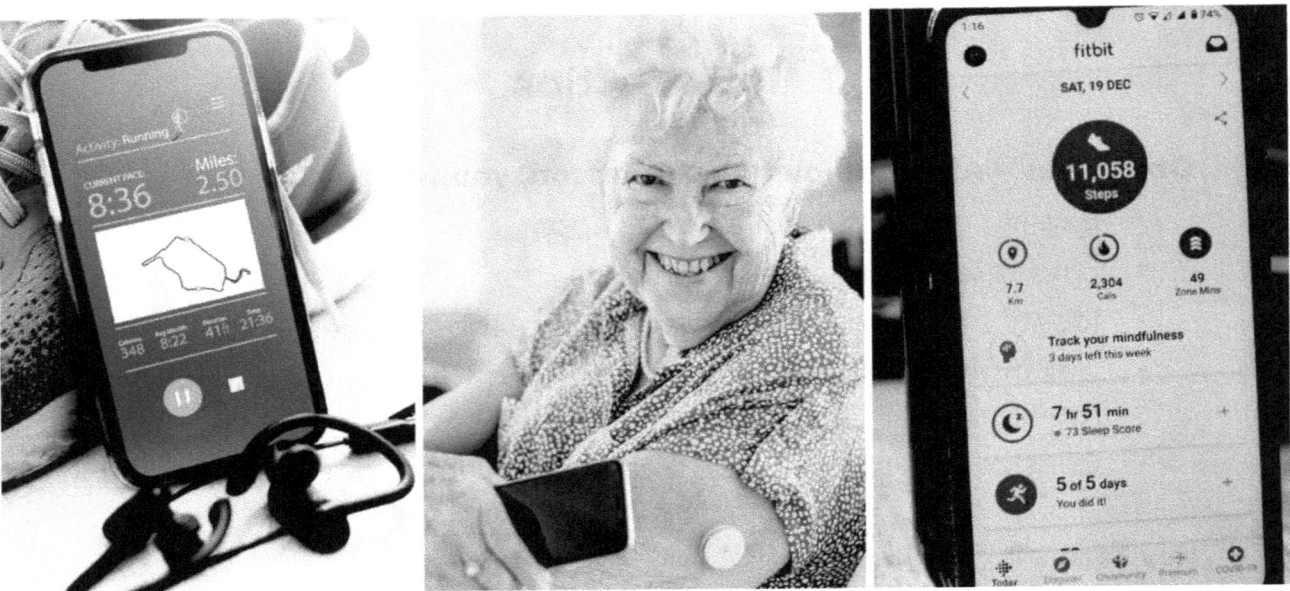

Technology is making it easier to monitor your health between visits to the doctor. In fact, there are mobile health apps available that help you eat better, stay on top of your health, and manage care routines. In Lesson One we defined a **mobile health app** as a software program used on a smartphone or tablet that helps you track your health, collect information, or talk with healthcare providers. Today there are countless health apps that expand access to information and encourage healthy behaviors.

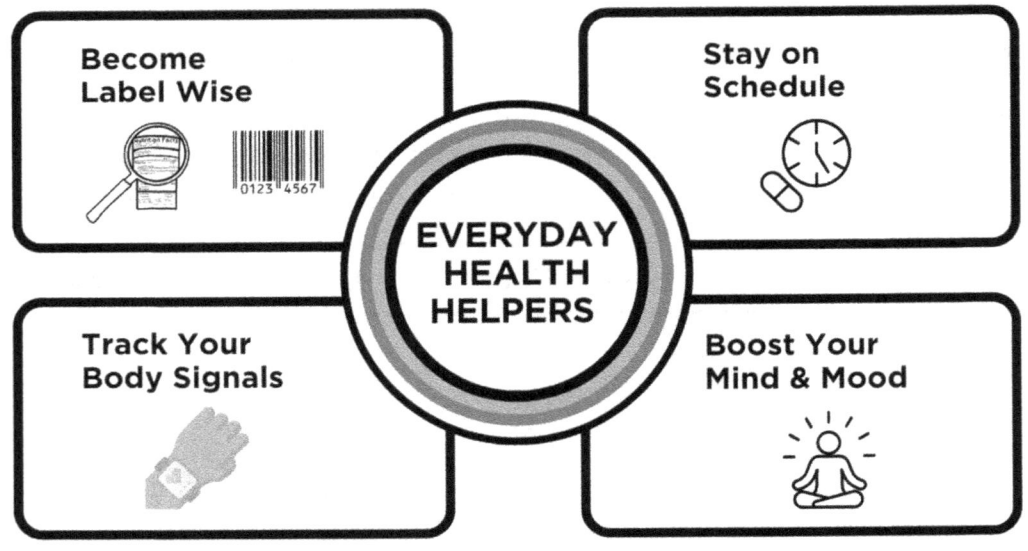

Figure 4-1: Achieve Your Health Goals with Apps

- **Become Label Wise** – These apps help you scan and read all types of labels. Whether it's your favorite bag of potato chips or the deodorant you use, you can check which options are healthier and make better choices about the food and personal care products you buy.
- **Track Your Body Signals** – Keeping track of your daily steps, sleep, heart rate, and blood pressure can help you stay in tune with your body and feel more prepared when you visit your doctor.
- **Stay on Schedule** – Apps can help you keep track of your medications, remind you when to take them, and when it's time to get refills.
- **Boost Your Mind & Mood** – Some apps are made to help with mental wellness. They can guide you to relax, breathe deeply, and feel recharged.

These goal-oriented categories and simple descriptions will help you find an app that matches your needs. Some apps may require wearable technology, or a wearable, like a watch, ring, or biosensor. As discussed in Lesson One, a **wearable** is a small device you wear on your body that helps track your health. A **biosensor** is a type of smart detector that measures heart rate, blood sugar, activity, and other body signals.

Apps That Work with Wearables	Apps That Don't Need a Wearable
These apps connect to a device you wear, like a smartwatch, fitness band, or biosensor. The wearable tracks your steps, heart rate, sleep, or other health numbers, and the app shows this information on your phone or tablet. **Examples:** • Apple Health app (integrates with Apple Watch) • Dexcom app (works with a continuous glucose monitor) • Oura app (works with the Oura ring)	These apps let you enter your own information (like weight, blood pressure, meals, or product barcode) directly into the app. They help you keep track of your health or check food and personal care choices without needing special devices. **Examples:** • MyFitnessPal (log meals and exercise) • Medisafe (set medication reminders) • Yuka (scan the barcode of food or personal care products)

A **continuous glucose monitor**, or CGM, is a tiny sensor that goes under the skin and checks blood sugar levels throughout the day. It is considered a type of biosensor.

Howie's How-Tos on Finding & Using Health Apps

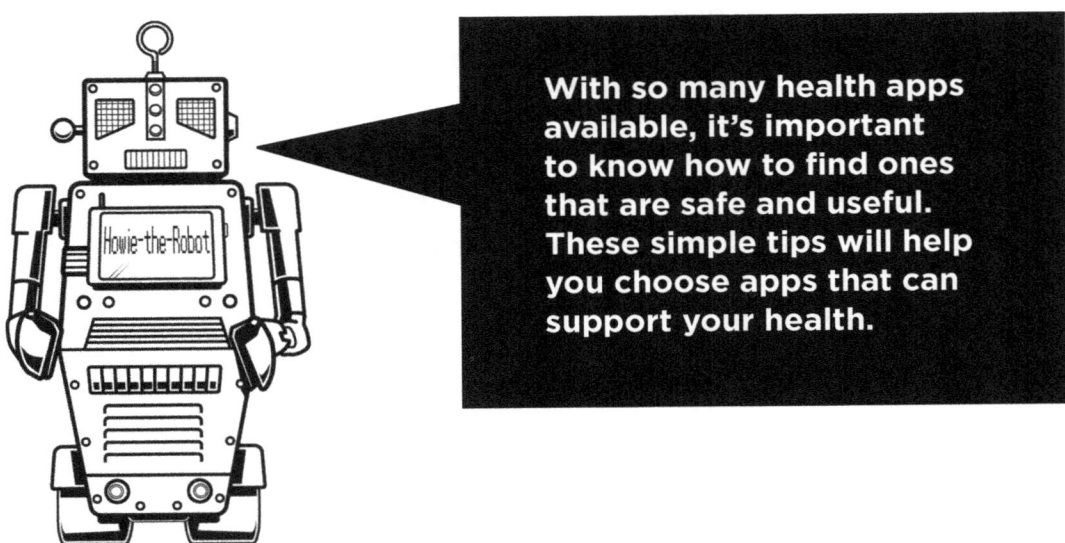

With so many health apps available, it's important to know how to find ones that are safe and useful. These simple tips will help you choose apps that can support your health.

1) **Use AI to help you search.** You can ask AI tools to suggest apps that match what you need. For example, you can type:

    "What are free apps that help track my sleep and are safe to use?"

    AI can give you a list to start with and help you know what to look for.

2) **Look for apps created by companies you trust.** These can include hospitals, health companies, well-known organizations, or referrals from trusted individuals. Generally, the app description will reveal who developed the app.

3) **Read reviews and ratings.** See what other people are saying. Choose apps with high ratings (4 stars or more) and positive reviews about ease of use and helpfulness.

4) **Look for privacy and safety information.** A good app should tell you how it keeps your sensitive health information safe. Look for words like "HIPAA-compliant" or "secure data."

5) **Start with free versions first.** Try free apps or free versions before paying for extra features. Many apps offer what you need at no cost.

6) **Ask a tech-for-care advocate, community health worker, or care manager.** If you're unsure, ask someone you trust who helps with digital health. They can suggest good options.

7) **Update your apps regularly.** Keep apps updated to make sure you have the latest features and security fixes.

Activity #1

Directions: Sara is using the Sugaroo™ app on her smartphone to help her think about how much sugar she is putting into her body. The app allows her to scan the barcode of her favorite foods and beverages and match the number of sugar cubes included in a serving for each item that she scans. One sugar cube equals roughly 4 grams of sugar.

Review the information below and help Sara match the correct number of sugar cubes with her favorite beverages, by writing the letter of the sugar cube picture under the drink that it matches. Then, answer the questions that follow.

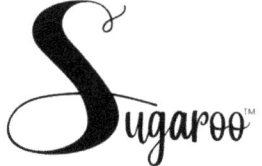

Daily Recommended Amount Sugar Cubes

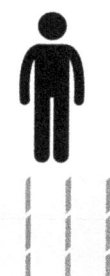

A	B	C	D
E	F	G	H

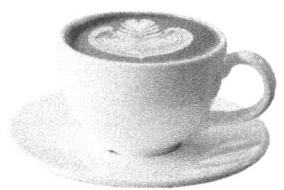
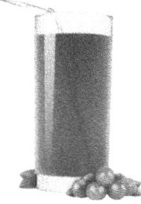
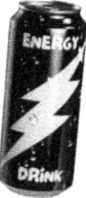
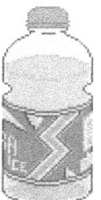

Cappuccino (12 grams) _____

Cranberry Juice (48 Grams) _____

Energy Drink (56 grams) _____

Sports Beverage (56 grams) _____

Pomegranate Juice   Root Beer   Soda   Orange Juice
(36 grams) _____   (44 Grams) _____   (48 grams) _____   (40 grams) _____

Kombucha
(28 grams) _____

Note: **Kombucha** is a fizzy drink made from tea and natural good bacteria that can help with digestion. Sugar content in beverages based on data from Avera Health and Global News.[2,3]

Questions:

1. Check the statements that are true.

   _____ Sara's favorite drinks, like soda and even fruit juice, add a lot of extra sugar to her diet.

   _____ If Sara drinks any two of her favorite beverages in the same day, she exceeds the daily recommended amount of sugar.

   _____ Drinking kombucha will allow Sara to stay below the recommended daily amount of sugar.

   _____ Drinking a cappuccino will allow Sara to stay below the recommended daily amount of sugar.

   _____ Based on the number of sugar cubes in her favorite drinks, Sara is putting very little sugar into her body.

   _____ If Sara keeps drinking her favorite sugary drinks often, she could increase her risk of getting diabetes over time.

2. What are some other drinks Sara can choose to help her cut down on sugar?

   _____

3. Based on the Sugaroo™ app, which of Sara's favorite drinks would you work to remove from your diet?

   _____

Remote Patient Monitoring

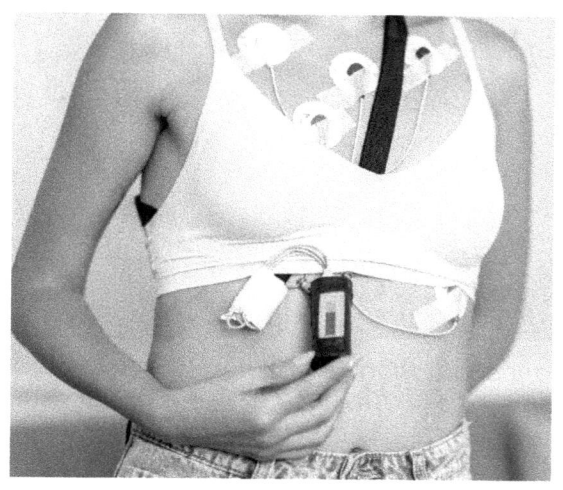

Technology now lets doctors check your health even when you're not at the doctor's office, clinic, or hospital. **Remote patient monitoring** uses tools like apps or devices to track heart rate, blood pressure, blood sugar and other vital signs from far away. **Vital signs** measure the body's most basic functions. The following table highlights some of the health data that can be tracked remotely and the indicators, or signals, care teams look for.

What can be tracked?	How measured?	Indicator	Healthy Range (Adults)
Body Temperature	Wearable sensors	Fever or infections	97°F – 99.1°F (36.1°C – 37.3°C) Source: Cleveland Clinic[4]
Blood Pressure	Wireless or cellular-connected blood pressure monitors	Heart health and stress levels	Less than 120/80 mmHg Source: American Heart Association[5]
Blood Sugar	Wearable devices like continuous glucose monitors	Energy and diabetes risk	70 – 99 mg/dL (fasting) Source: American Diabetes Association[6]
Heart Rate	Smartwatches, chest straps, and other wearables	How fast, or slow, your heart beats	60 – 100 beats per minute (resting) Source: Mayo Clinic[7]
Oxygen Saturation	Pulse oximeter	How *well* you breathe	95% – 100% Source: Mayo Clinic[8]
Respiratory Rate	Devices that detect chest wall movements or breathing	How *often* you breathe	12 – 20 breaths per minute Source: American CPR Care Association[9]
Patient-Reported Outcomes (PROs)	Text messaging, web-based platforms or forms, mobile apps	How you feel each day	Outcomes will vary

Most remote patient monitoring systems require an internet connection — either Wi-Fi or cell service — to send your health information to your doctor. For example, measuring **oxygen saturation**, which tracks how much oxygen is in the blood and shows how well the lungs are working to get oxygen into the body, relies on a connected pulse oximeter. The **pulse oximeter** clips onto your finger and sends a blood oxygen reading and heart rate through the internet directly to the doctor or nurse. As a result, the care team is able to catch problems early, especially for people with breathing issues like asthma or COPD (chronic obstructive pulmonary disease). **COPD** is a condition caused by damage to the airways.

Patients can also use remote patient monitoring systems to describe and report symptoms, providing a more complete picture of their health. Good reports might include things like feeling no pain, being in a good mood, or walking every day. On the other hand, responses like "still having pain," "feeling tired or sad," or "not able to walk as usual" help care teams know when more support or a change in care is needed.

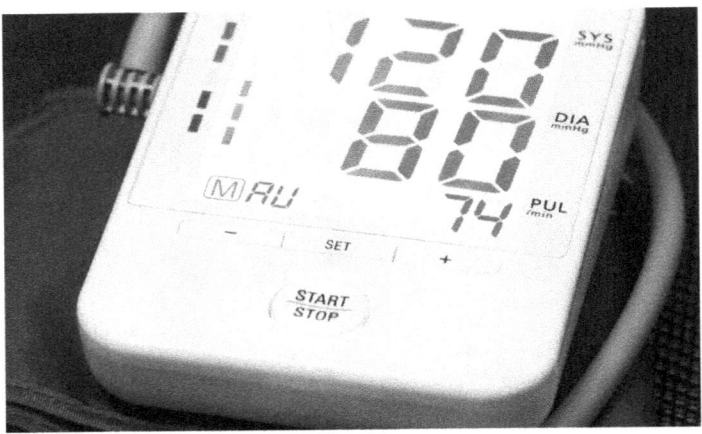

Connected Blood Pressure Monitor

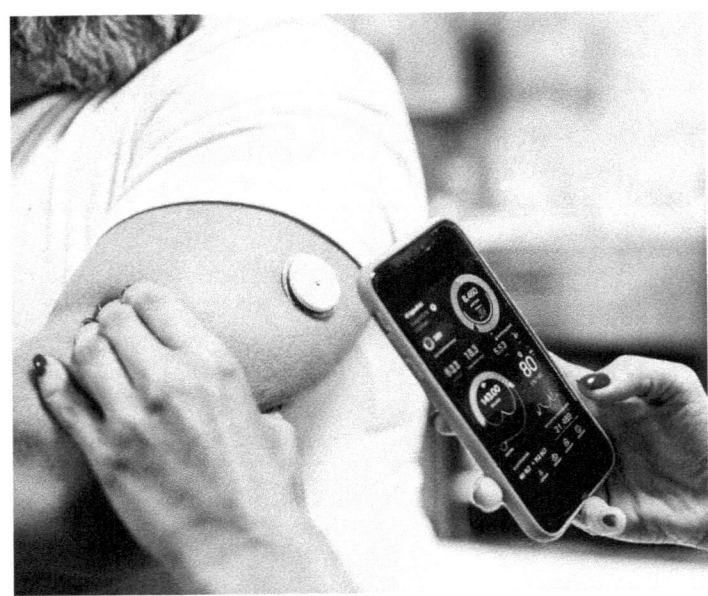

Continuous Glucose Monitor

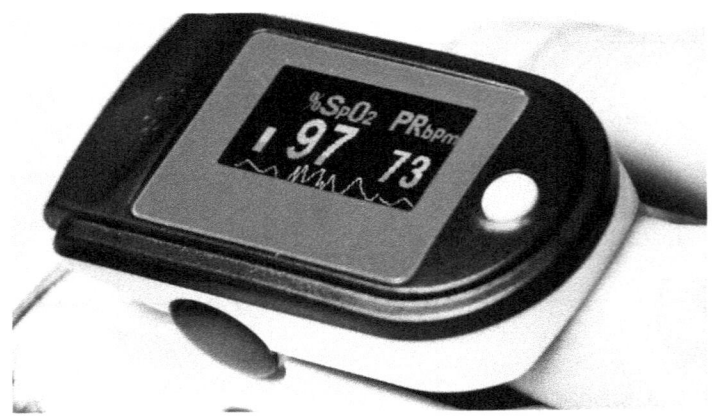

Pulse Oximeter

Activity #2

Directions: Read each question and provide the **best** answer.

1. What is the primary purpose of remote patient monitoring?

    A) To find top-rated local clinics

    B) To communicate with your care team

    C) To track weight loss

    D) To track health signs and share them with your doctor

2. Which of the following is *not* a vital sign that is usually checked during remote patient monitoring?

    A) Blood pressure

    B) Oxygen level

    C) Eye color

    D) Heart rate

3. Why is it helpful to send your health data to your doctor between visits?

    A) It replaces the need for future appointments.

    B) It helps the doctor better understand your health and choose the right treatment plan.

    C) It saves you time and money.

    D) The quality of care is better than in-person visits.

4. What can a body temperature of 101°F (38.3°C) tell your doctor?

    A) You are drinking enough water.

    B) You may have an infection.

    C) You need more sleep.

    D) You are hungry.

5. Why is it helpful to know your respiratory rate?

    A) To check if you're breathing normally

    B) To help count your daily steps

    C) To track your eating habits

    D) To improve your eyesight

6. What is a Patient-Reported Outcome (PRO)?

    A) A lab result

    B) A number from your smartwatch

    C) A message from your doctor

    D) How you say you feel

7. Which of the following shows a good PRO report?

    A) "I'm very dizzy and confused."

    B) "I didn't take my medicine this week."

    C) "No pain today. I walked 20 minutes."

    D) "I skipped breakfast and lunch."

8. **True** or **False**. Write **T** for True or **F** for False next to the statements below.

    _____ a) A normal resting heart rate is the same for everyone.

    _____ b) If your PRO report says "feeling tired all day" for many days in a row, your care team should know.

The R.E.E.L.

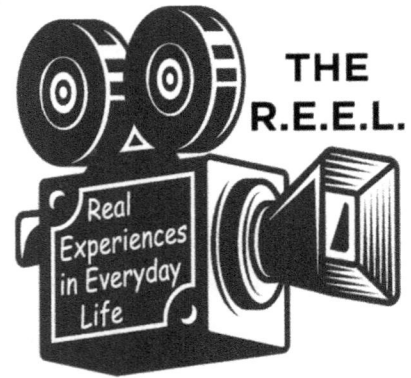

Aging in Place

Many older adults struggle with aging in place, or staying in their home as they age. They often worry about having no one to care for them and not wanting to be a burden on family and friends. There's a better, more empowered way to think about staying healthy and independent at home.

Directions: Imagine you want to stay in your home as you get older. If it makes sense for your health and finances, you'll need your circle of care (remember Lesson One) — and some helpful tools — to keep you safe, healthy, and connected.

Consider each situation and circle the "Care Help" that best applies to you.

Situation	Care Help (Circle all that apply, or write your own under "Other")			
1) You want reminders to take your medicine every day.	A. Care Coordinator	B. Family	C. Mobile Health App	D. Other ___
2) You feel sad and lonely and want someone to talk to.	A. Friend	B. Therapist	C. Community Health Worker	D. Other ___
3) You don't understand your lab results in the patient portal.	A. Care Coordinator	B. Nurse	C. AI Tool like ChatGPT	D. Other ___

Circle a tool below that you currently use or would consider using. Explain how it could help you or someone you know stay independent.

Patient Portal   Video Visits   Mobile Apps   Smartwatch   AI Chatbot

<u>Note:</u> An **AI chatbot** is a computer program or virtual assistant that can talk with you, answer questions, and help you find information.

___

___

Aging in place doesn't mean going it alone. It means building the right team, using the right tools, and speaking up when you need help.

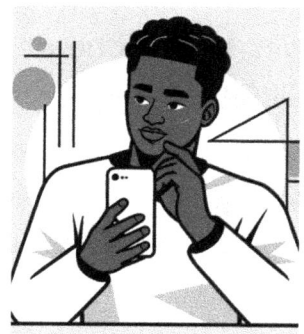

Show What You Know!

Congratulations on completing the lesson. You've made great progress. Enter your site code and the information below to answer a few quick questions about what you learned.

Lesson Four	Checkpoint Number: **8**

Key Terms

Aging In Place	Staying in your home as you age.
AI Chatbot	A computer program that can talk with you, answer questions, and help you find information.
Biosensor	A type of smart detector that measures heart rate, blood sugar, activity, and other body signals.
Continuous Glucose Monitor	A tiny sensor that goes under the skin and checks blood sugar levels throughout the day.
COPD	A condition caused by damage to the airways.
Kombucha	A fizzy drink made from tea and natural good bacteria that can help with digestion.
Mobile Health App	A software program used on a smartphone or tablet that helps you track your health.
Oxygen Saturation	Tracks how much oxygen is in the blood and shows how well the lungs are working to get oxygen into the body.
Patient-Reported Outcome	How you say you feel and the experience you report.
Pulse Oximeter	A medical device that tracks how much oxygen is in the blood.
Remote Patient Monitoring	Uses tools like apps or devices to track heart rate, blood pressure, blood sugar and other vital signs from far away.
Vital Signs	Measure the body's most basic functions.
Wearable	A small device you wear on your body that helps track your health.

LESSON FIVE: Trusting Health Information

Introduction

Objectives – After completing this lesson, you will be able to:
- Describe health misinformation
- Spot propaganda, cognitive bias, and trigger words
- Use the CLEAR framework to test and respond to health information
- Create AI prompts for fact-finding

Key Terms
- CLEAR Head Approach
- Cognitive Bias
- Health Misinformation
- Microplastics
- Opioid Drugs
- Propaganda
- Trigger Words
- Voice-Activated Speaker

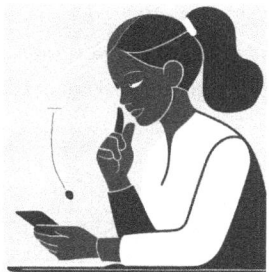

Let's Get Started!

Your voice matters. Enter your site code and the information below to share what you already know and what you hope to learn about trusting health information.

| Lesson Five | Checkpoint Number: **9** |

Health Misinformation

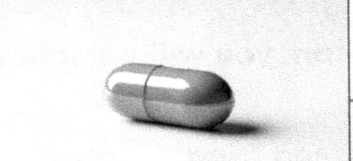
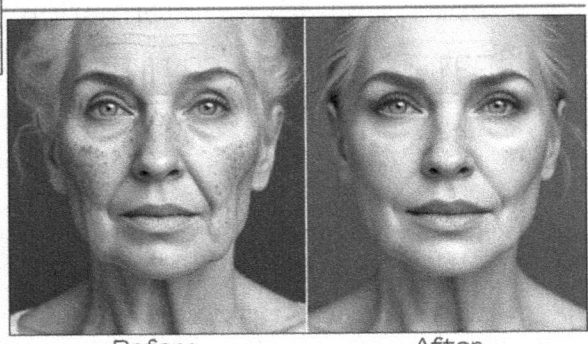

Fictional Ad

Health misinformation is false or misleading health information that can cause confusion or harm if people believe it. Unfortunately, misleading health messages can come from websites, social media, and traditional media spaces that sound trustworthy but are not accurate. Traditional media spaces include print advertisements similar to the one featured above, magazine articles, television news segments, and radio talk shows.

You might also, without meaning to, spread health misinformation. For example, as someone who uses social media, you might see a large number of posts and videos each day. If you share something that's misleading or false — without checking first — you can accidentally help spread it. This often happens because of mental shortcuts — quick ways our brain processes information that can lead to mistakes in judgment. These shortcuts, called **cognitive biases**, are patterns in thinking that can cause people to believe or share something without having all the facts.

Health misinformation can also come in the form of propaganda and fear. **Propaganda** is when health information is shared to push a certain belief or agenda, often using emotions instead of balanced facts. For example, an ad for a weight-loss supplement might only show dramatic "before and after" photos without sharing that the results came from surgery, not the pill.

Fear is used to scare people into making a quick choice instead of helping them make an informed one. References to death, disease, outbreak, and mayhem can grab attention and steer public opinion. Cognitive bias, propaganda, and fear are triggers that drive behavior, and in some instances, lead to rash decision-making.

Cognitive Bias	Propaganda	Fear
You start taking a "miracle vitamin" because you see dozens of friends posting about it online, even though you've never checked if it's safe or effective.	"This product is endorsed by celebrities, so you know it works!"	"Your health will fail quickly unless you buy this supplement today."

Howie's How-Tos on Spotting Fear & Propaganda

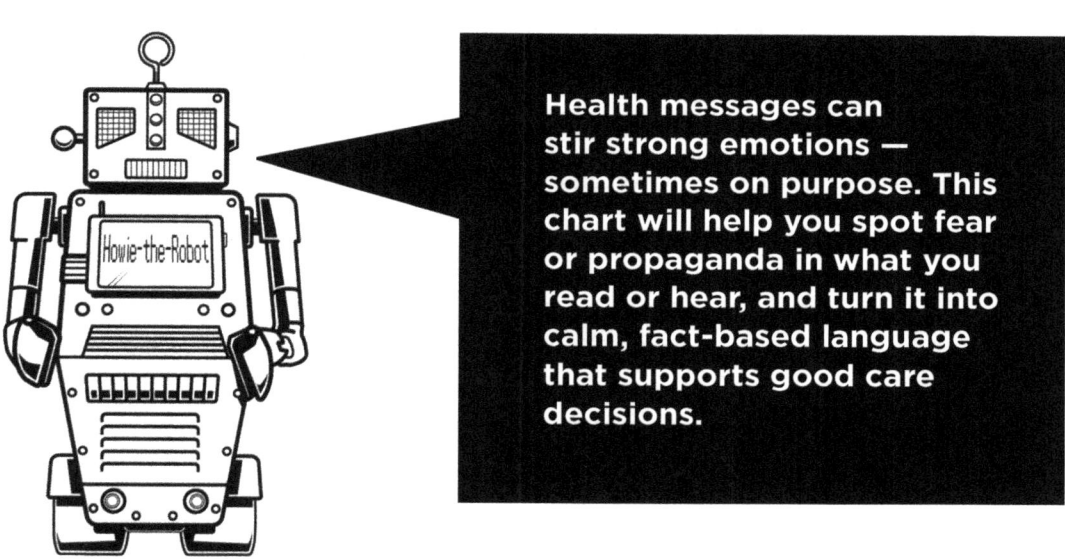

Health messages can stir strong emotions — sometimes on purpose. This chart will help you spot fear or propaganda in what you read or hear, and turn it into calm, fact-based language that supports good care decisions.

Fear/Propaganda Message	Trigger	Fact-Based Switch
"You are at serious risk unless you act now!"	Urgency and danger	"Talk with your care team to understand your personal risk and options."

Fear/Propaganda Message	Trigger	Fact-Based Switch
"Everyone in your area is getting sick from this!"	Overgeneralization	"Recent reports show cases in some areas. Check reliable local health data for accurate numbers."
"This new pill will save your life instantly!"	Miracle cure	"Ask your provider about the pill's benefits, risks, and research before deciding."

When faced with propaganda or messages of fear, be sure to ask yourself if a trustworthy source can confirm how big this risk really is. Also, be sure to see if other reliable sources agree with the claim. Before making a decision, ask a few questions to assess how accurate the information is.

- Who is sharing this information, and can they be trusted?
- What evidence or facts support the claim?
- Does this match what I've learned from my doctor, nurse, or experienced firsthand — or does it sound very different?
- Am I letting fear of the worst outcome stop me from thinking clearly?

Activity #1

Directions: Read each scenario and identify the emotional trigger as either cognitive bias, propaganda, or fear. Circle the **best** answer.

1. Heather reads the following social media ad: *"Join the wellness revolution now! Everyone is doing it — don't be left out."* Heather doesn't want to miss out so she signs up and becomes a member.

    Cognitive Bias   Propaganda   Fear

2. Martin believes a certain herbal tea cures colds, so he only reads articles and watches videos that say it works, while ignoring research that shows no benefit.

    Cognitive Bias   Propaganda   Fear

3. Eddie and Sam are miners who work in underground tunnels. Sam goes to a local sauna each week and wants Eddie to join him. He says the following to Eddie: "If you don't detox soon, your body will be full of dangerous toxins."

    Cognitive Bias   Propaganda   Fear

4. After hearing about a rare side effect from a friend's mammogram, Michelle believes it's very common, even though data shows it almost never happens. She decides to cancel her upcoming appointment and schedule her mammogram for next year.

    Cognitive Bias   Propaganda   Fear

5. As Kyle prepares to watch his favorite podcast, he sees an ad that claims that eating a certain food will ruin his health forever. It just so happens that Kyle eats this food on a regular basis and decides to click the link to learn more.

    Cognitive Bias   Propaganda   Fear

6. Beverly wants to get healthier and has a goal of losing at least 20 pounds. She hears her favorite talk show host talk about a certain diet that "guarantees" fast results. This claim stays in her mind, even after her doctor explains there is no proof it works. Beverly decides to try the diet anyway.

    Cognitive Bias   Propaganda   Fear

7. Travis went to his local clinic after hurting his knee. The waiting room was full because many people were being treated for overdoses from a "bad batch" of **opioid drugs** (strong painkillers that can be very addictive). The next day on the news, a politician said the city's drug problem was under control and there was no reason to worry.

    Cognitive Bias   Propaganda   Fear

8. Sergio has type 2 diabetes and sees this online ad described in the photo. He carefully considers purchasing the "breakthrough pill" for himself.

    Cognitive Bias

    Propaganda

    Fear

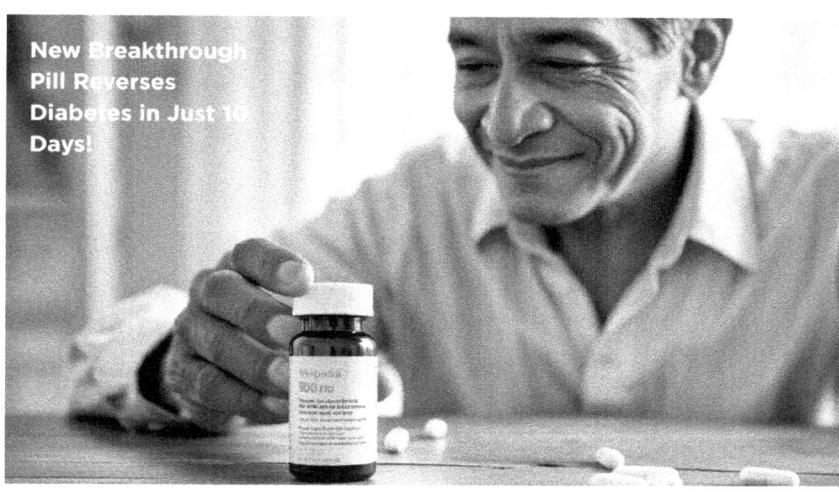

9. What is the reason for your choice in Scenario #8?

_____

_____

CLEAR Head Approach

When it comes to health information, it's easy to be influenced by strong emotions, convincing stories, or flashy headlines. Developing a practice of recognizing cognitive bias, propaganda, and fear, and verifying facts before sharing, leads to health choices that are safer and more effective. Everyone can build this habit themselves and avoid quick-fix claims and other health traps.

The **CLEAR** Framework™, or CLEAR Head Approach™ (CLEAR), helps you slow down, cool your feelings, and think carefully before acting on health information. By practicing CLEAR, you build the habit of making calmer, evidence-based choices about your health.

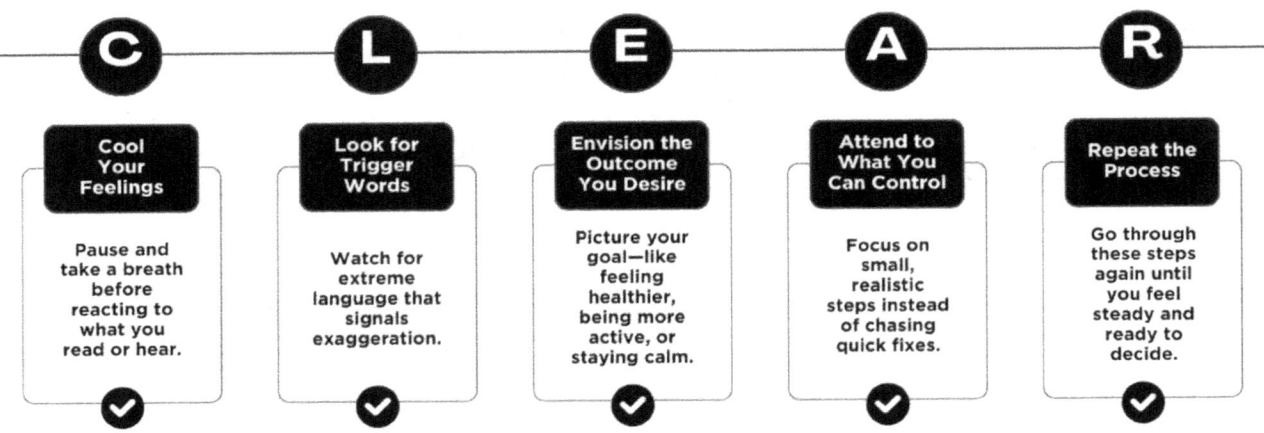

It is important to remember that strong emotions like fear, anger, and hatred can cloud judgment. Also, **trigger words** like *always, never, everyone, nothing,* and *nobody* are often used on purpose to influence behavior. Using CLEAR regularly can help you stay aware and steady, even when health challenges come your way. It reminds you to test automatic thoughts, focus on what you can control, and make smart choices with a calm, clear mind.

Activity #2

Directions: Read each question and provide the **best** answer.

1. Identify all the trigger words, or phrases, in the following advertisement.

    "Erase every wrinkle instantly with our miracle injection! Look 20 years younger in just one week — guaranteed. Unlike anything you've ever seen, this perfect treatment gives you flawless, youthful skin that lasts forever. Everyone will notice your transformation, and you'll never feel old again."

    _____

    _____

2. **Microplastics** are tiny pieces of plastic that break down from bottles, bags, and other plastic products. They are so small you usually can't see them, but they can end up in food, water, and even the air.[10]

    A well-known online influencer makes a claim about microplastics, as shown below. Identify all the trigger words, or phrases, that sound extreme or designed to scare you.

    "Everyone who drinks bottled water is filling their body with deadly microplastics! These tiny plastic pieces, smaller than a grain of sand, are invading your organs and causing cancer in millions of people. No one is safe — every sip adds poison to your system. Stop drinking bottled water now, before it's too late!"

    _____

    _____

3. Review the words you identified in the first two questions. How do they make the claims more emotional than factual?

    _____

    _____

    _____

4. What real evidence would you need to check before believing either claim?

_____

_____

5. Norman's doctor tells him that his blood pressure is very high and provides a treatment plan, which includes medication, cutting back on salty foods, and walking 20 minutes each day. Norman shares the news with his wife and tells her that given his luck, he will "probably have a stroke tomorrow."

Apply the CLEAR Framework (CLEAR Head Approach) to help Norman make smart choices with a calm, clear mind.

C	a) How can Norman cool his feelings?
L	b) What trigger words did Norman use to jump to the worst possible outcome?
E	c) How can Norman envision a positive health outcome?
A	d) How can Norman attend to what he can control?
R	e) What can Norman do if his mind jumps to worst case thinking?

AI for Fact-Finding

AI can be a helpful tool for checking health information. It is very good at quickly scanning, comparing, and explaining large amounts of information. Here's how:

1) **Scanning**. AI can quickly scan articles, websites, or reports and point out where the information comes from, making it easier to judge if a source is trustworthy.

2) **Comparing**. AI can compare different sources, so you can see if experts agree or if there are warning signs of misinformation.

3) **Explaining**. AI can turn confusing medical terms into plain language that's easier to understand. It can also break down statistics, helping explain what the numbers really mean. For example, if you hear "80% of people improved after treatment," AI can help check whether the study had enough people to make that number matter. This way, you can see if statistics are being used in a helpful way — or if they're being used to mislead.

Confusing Medical Term	AI → Quick Definition	AI → Plain Explanation
BMI (Body Mass Index)	"A number that shows if your weight is healthy for your height."	"Doctors use BMI to see if someone is underweight, at a healthy weight, overweight, or obese. It doesn't measure body fat directly, so it doesn't always tell the full story, but it gives a quick picture of health."
Anemia	"Low iron in the blood."	"Your body doesn't have enough healthy red blood cells to carry oxygen. This can make you feel tired, weak, or dizzy."

<u>Note:</u> AI responses are from ChatGPT and are at a 5th grade level.

More on Statistics

People who quit smoking reduce their risk of lung cancer by about **50% after 10 years** compared to those who keep smoking.

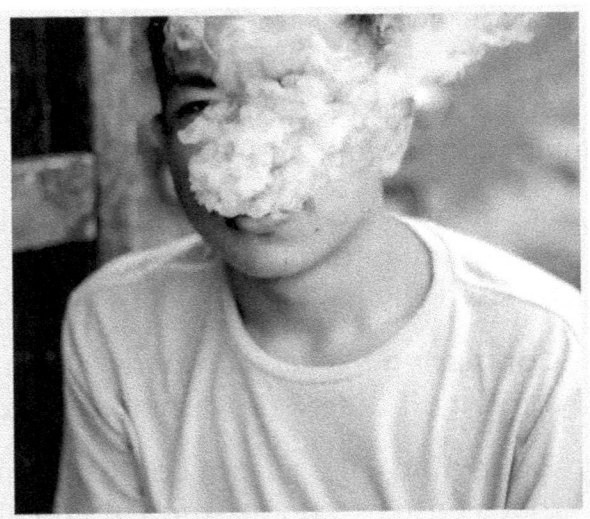

Using AI to Investigate the "Quit Smoking" Claim

- **Sample AI Prompt (1):** Share the claim along with the following question: Is there good long-term proof from trusted sources to support this claim?

- **AI Response (1):** "Yes. Many long-term studies from trusted sources, like the American Cancer Society and the National Cancer Institute, show that quitting smoking lowers the risk of lung cancer. The longer a person stays smoke-free, the more their risk drops — sometimes close to the level of someone who never smoked."

- **Sample AI Prompt (2):** Based on this response, what question should I ask my doctor?

- **AI Response (2):** "Based on my health history, how much can quitting smoking lower my risk of lung cancer, and how long would it take to see real benefits?"

Benefits of AI for Fact-Finding:

1) **Quick Helper for Testing Health Claims.** AI can quickly scan information so you don't have to start from scratch.

2) **Helps You Spot and Compare Sources.** It can show where the information comes from and how sources line up.

3) **Turns Numbers into Questions.** AI can explain statistics and help you ask, "Does this apply to me?"

4) **Gives You Plain Language for Your Care Team.** It can turn confusing medical terms into words you can use when talking to your doctor or nurse.

5) **Builds Your Confidence in Your Health Decisions**. By practicing with AI, you feel more in control of your choices.

Risks of AI for Fact-Finding:

1) **Wrong or Incomplete Answers**. AI can sometimes give information that sounds right, but is actually wrong or missing important details.
   → Risk Prompt: "How do I know if this AI answer is complete and based on trusted sources?"

2) **Bias in the Information.** AI may reflect the same mistakes or biases that exist in the data it was trained on.
   → Risk Prompt: "Could this AI answer be showing bias or only one side of the story?"

3) **Lack of Personal Context.** AI does not know your personal health history or life experiences, so answers may not apply to your specific situation.
   → Risk Prompt: "What follow-up question should I ask my doctor to see if this information fits my case?"

4) **Outdated Information:** AI may give health answers based on old sources that no longer match the latest medical research.
   → Risk Prompt: "Is this information current, or should I check with a trusted source for the latest guidance?"

Bottom Line: AI is a helpful tool for making sense of health claims and numbers, but it should support — not replace — your own judgment and your care team's advice.

The R.E.E.L.

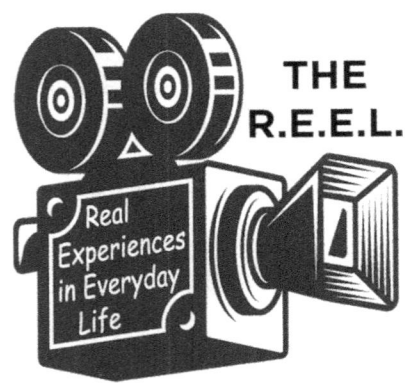

Voice Use for AI Fact-Finding

Speaking your prompt can be easier and faster than typing — especially when you're busy or on the go. Using the microphone on your device or a **voice-activated speaker** lets you ask health questions out loud, just like you would with your doctor or nurse.

  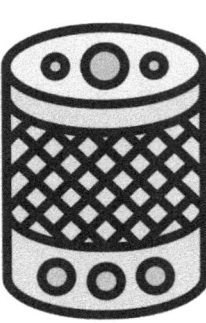

Scenario: Joel is a medical assistant who works at a local clinic. He sees patients with low literacy, vision problems, and limited typing skills. He wants to know how encouraging the use of voice tools for AI fact-finding can lead to more meaningful, two-way conversations with these patients.

Based on your knowledge, what response will you share with Joel?

_____

_____

_____

_____

Activity #3

Directions: Read each scenario and write an AI fact-finding prompt (question you would ask) to help make sense of the situation.

Scenario 1: Vicky and Sam's Son Zack

Vicky and Sam's son, Zack, is in first grade. His teacher says Zack has a hard time finishing his work and paying attention. He also has trouble sitting still in class. The school nurse thinks it could be ADHD and even mentions that Zack might need medicine called a stimulant. She reminds them to see a doctor for a second opinion. Before the appointment, Vicky and Sam want to use AI to look up facts so they can ask better questions and understand what's really going on.

_____

_____

_____

Scenario 2: Understanding a Measles Outbreak

Natasha lives in a small rural county. Recently, there has been a measles outbreak affecting her community and a region of roughly 650,000 people. So far, there have been 700 cases, 100 hospitalizations, and 2 deaths. The local news is reporting on the outbreak nonstop, and it feels overwhelming. Natasha wants to use AI to make sense of the numbers so she can understand how serious the outbreak is and come up with better questions to ask her doctor or public health officials.

_____

_____

_____

Scenario 3: Reading Food Labels

Tyrone is looking at the label on one of his favorite snack foods. He sees that the ingredients list includes monosodium glutamate (MSG) and some artificial colors called Yellow 6, Yellow 5, and Red 40. Tyrone isn't sure what these ingredients are or if they are safe to eat. He decides to use AI to look up reliable information so that he can ask better questions when he talks with a nutritionist.

_____

_____

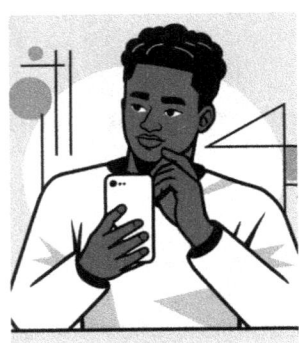

Show What You Know!

Congratulations on completing the lesson. You've made great progress. Enter your site code and the information below to answer a few quick questions about what you learned.

| Lesson Five | Checkpoint Number: **10** |

Key Terms

CLEAR Head Approach	A five-step framework developed by author Angela Harris to help you slow down, cool your feelings, and think carefully before acting.
Cognitive Bias	A pattern in thinking that can cause people to believe or share something without having all the facts.
Health Misinformation	False or misleading health information that can cause confusion or harm if people believe it.
Microplastics	Tiny plastic pieces, smaller than a grain of sand.
Opioid Drugs	Strong painkillers that can be very addictive.
Propaganda	When health information is shared to push a certain belief or agenda, often using emotions instead of balanced facts.
Trigger Words	Words like always, never, everyone, nothing, nobody, and perfect used on purpose to influence behavior.
Voice-Activated Speaker	A device you can talk to that answers questions or does tasks when you speak.

LESSON SIX: Protecting Health Information

Introduction

Objectives – After completing this lesson, you will be able to:

- Explain patient rights under the Health Insurance Portability and Accountability Act (HIPAA)
- Identify a phishing scam
- Create a strong password
- Protect yourself from healthcare fraud
- Practice using two-factor authentication
- Recognize when your protected health information (PHI) is not being kept safe and private

Key Terms

- Care Operations
- Diagnosis
- Healthcare Fraud
- HIPAA
- Notice of Privacy Practices (NPP)
- Orthodontist
- Phishing Scam
- Security Awareness Training
- Two-Factor Authentication

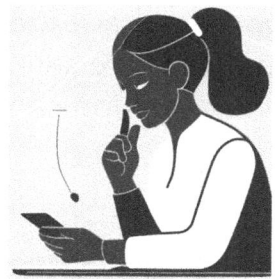

Let's Get Started!

Your voice matters. Enter your site code and the information below to share what you already know and what you hope to learn about protecting health information.

| Lesson Six | Checkpoint Number: **11** |

Patient Rights

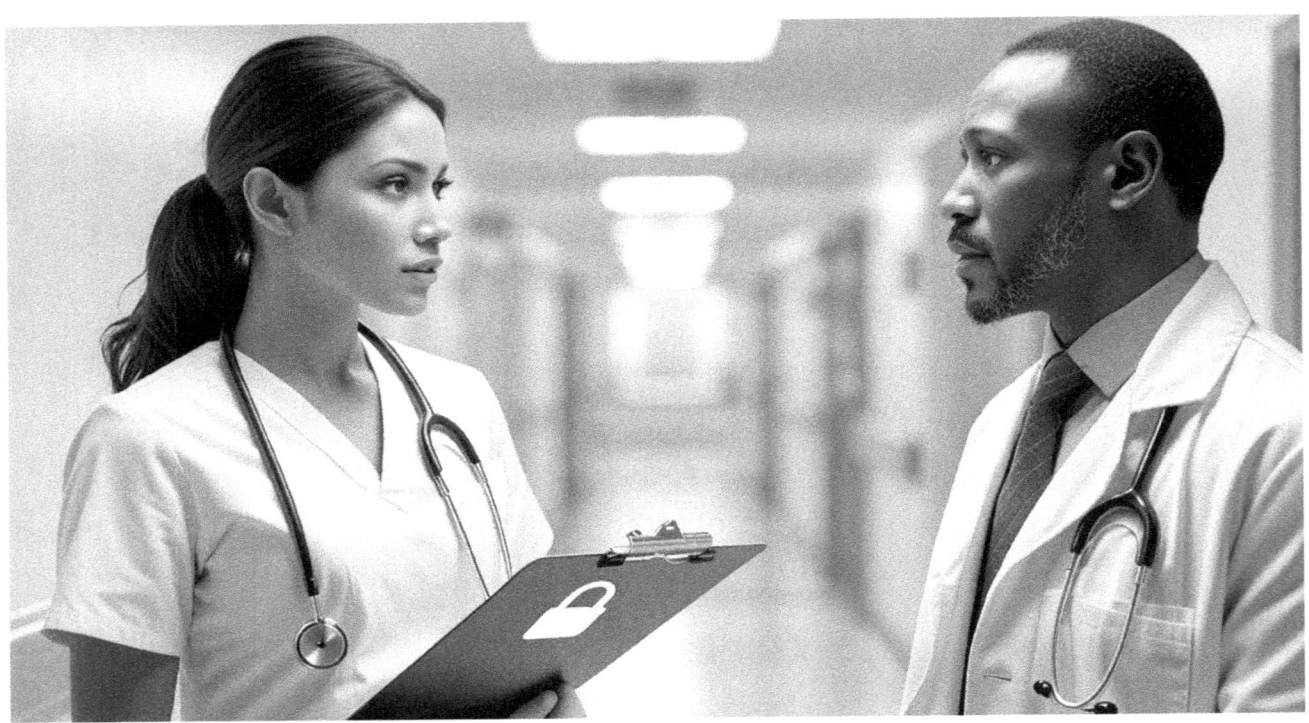

As discussed in Lesson Three, the Health Insurance Portability and Accountability Act, or **HIPAA**, is a law that protects your personal health information and makes sure doctors, nurses, and clinics keep it private and secure. HIPAA gives you the right to keep your health information private, to see and get copies of your medical records, and to know who has shared your information.

In a digital environment, your provider can share your information only when it is needed for treatment, payment, or care operations. **Care operations** are the behind-the-scenes activities that clinics and hospitals do to make patient care safe, organized, and better. The next examples show how private health information can be shared in everyday situations.

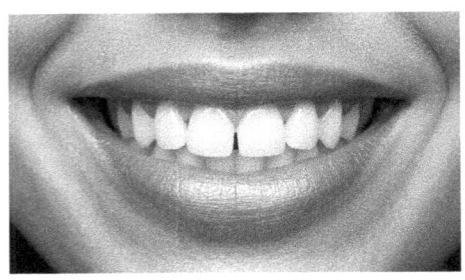

Treatment

Situation:

Maria's dentist sends her X-rays to an **orthodontist** to see how her teeth and jaws are positioned. An orthodontist is a type of dentist who is trained to fix crooked teeth and jaws, often by using braces or clear aligners.

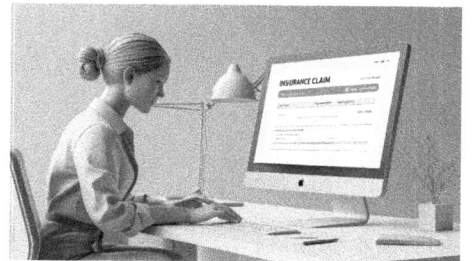
Payment

Situation:
The medical billing specialist sends information about your visit to your insurance company so the bill can be paid.

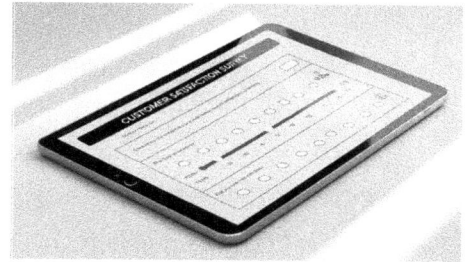
Care Operations

Situation:
A clinic uses your customer satisfaction survey to review how well they are caring for people and to find ways to improve.

Knowing your rights about your health information is important because it helps you decide who can see it, protects your privacy, and makes sure you are treated fairly and with respect. The following table summarizes some of the rights you have as a patient.

Right	Example
1) Right to See Your Records	You can look at your health records and ask for a copy. You can also have them sent to another person you trust.
2) Right to Fix Mistakes	If something in your health record is wrong or missing, you can ask to have it corrected.
3) Right to Know How Your Information Is Used	You must be given a written notice that explains how your health information may be shared. This notice is called a **notice of privacy practices**, or NPP.
4) Right to Ask for Limits	You can ask your doctor not to share your health information for certain reasons, like payment or office tasks, but the doctor doesn't always have to agree.

Activity #1

Directions: Read each question. Circle the **best** answer.

1. Which of the following is a right patients have under HIPAA?

    A) The right to have personal protective equipment (PPE) like KN95 masks in the waiting room for their use.

    B) The right to get a copy of their medical records and share them with someone they trust.

    C) The right to choose which staff member takes their blood pressure.

    D) The right to question the accuracy of a bill.

2. Which of the following is an example of how HIPAA protects patient privacy?

    A) A hospital lets a patient choose the time they would like to bathe.

    B) A patient is told they can't eat or drink before a surgery.

    C) A nurse explains to a patient that their lab results will only be shared with doctors involved in their care.

    D) A clinic posts everyone's test results on a bulletin board so staff can see them.

3. Which of the following is not an example of care operations?

    A) Training staff on how to grow in their jobs or move into new roles.

    B) Reviewing charts to make sure treatments are safe and follow best practices.

    C) Looking at data to find ways to shorten wait times or improve patient care.

    D) Checking patient records to see if people are getting needed screenings.

4. Jamal notices his medical record says he is allergic to penicillin, but he is not. He asks the clinic to correct it. Which right is Jamal exercising?

    A) Right to See His Records

    B) Right to Fix Mistakes

    C) Right to Know How His Information is Used

    D) Right to Ask for Limits

5. Freddie tells his doctor not to share information about his therapy sessions with his insurance company. The doctor listens, but explains they may not always be able to agree. Which right is Freddie using?

    A) Right to See His Records

    B) Right to Fix Mistakes

    C) Right to Know How His Information is Used

    D) Right to Ask for Limits

6. Before her first visit, Gloria receives a paper that explains how the clinic may share her health information. Which right is Gloria using?

    A) Right to See Her Records

    B) Right to Fix Mistakes

    C) Right to Know How Her Information is Used

    D) Right to Ask for Limits

7. Teresa asks her clinic for a copy of her lab results so she can bring them to a specialist. Which right is Teresa asking for?

    A) Right to See Her Records

    B) Right to Fix Mistakes

    C) Right to Know How Her Information is Used

    D) Right to Ask for Limits

8. Tom sees that his medical record says he takes a weight-loss drug, but he has never been prescribed it, so he asks to have it corrected. Which right is Tom asking for?

    A) Right to See His Records

    B) Right to Fix Mistakes

    C) Right to Know How His Information is Used

    D) Right to Ask for Limits

Patient Responsibilities

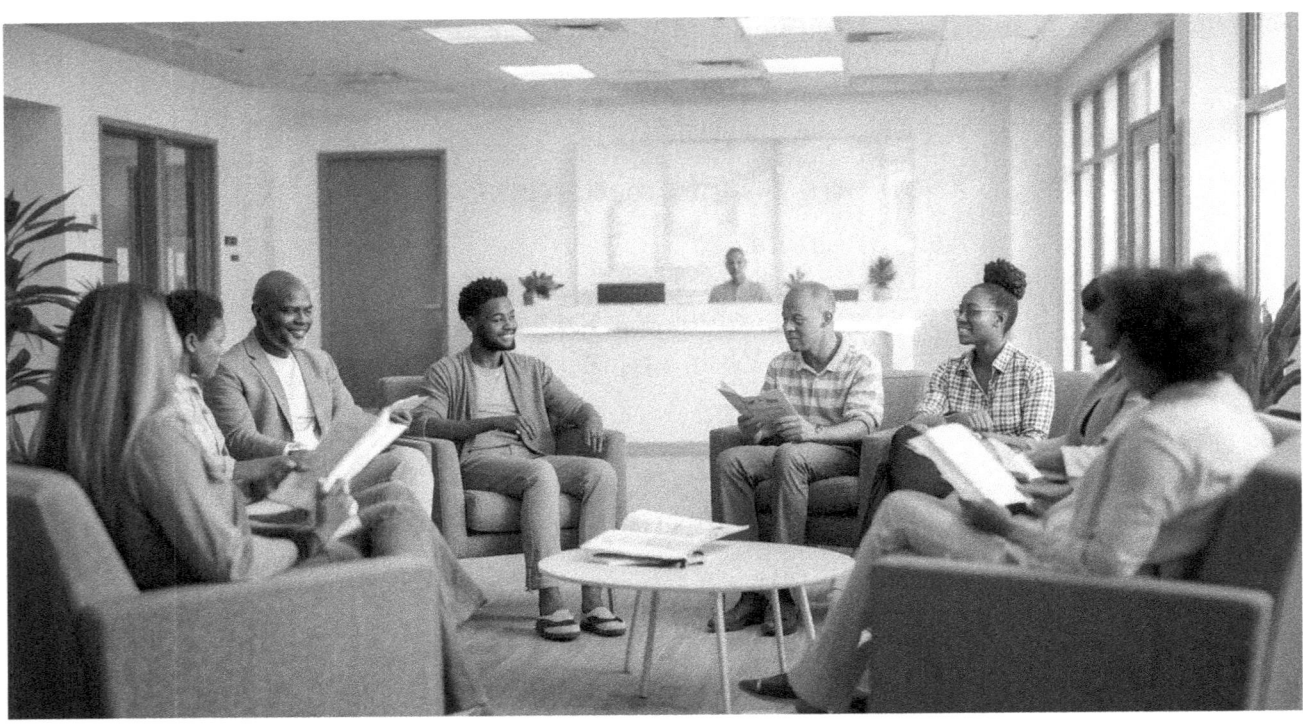

Just like doctors and nurses must protect your health information, patients also have an important role to play. By using strong passwords, turning on two-factor authentication, and being careful with scams, you can help keep your personal information safe.

Knowing how to protect sensitive health data can be a challenge for many individuals, as bad actors use a variety of schemes to take advantage of unknowing victims. **Security awareness training** helps prevent these tricks by teaching you how to spot online threats, protect your accounts, and keep sensitive information safe. Think of this section as a crash course in security awareness.

Suspicious Emails

Questions: Consider the following two emails. Can you tell which one is safe and which one is a scam? What red flags appear in the scam email?

_____

_____

_____

Figure 6-1: Main Street Clinic

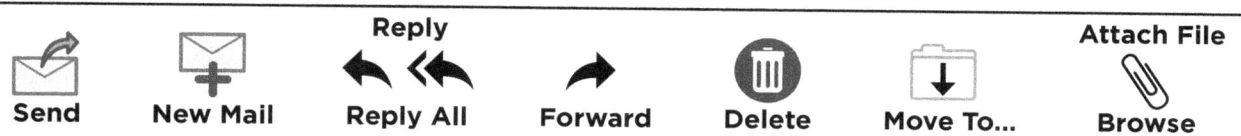

Email Folders	From:	Main Street Clinic
Inbox Drafts Sent Deleted Items Junk Email Contacts	Subject:	Important: Verify Your Account Now!
	Message:	Dear Patient, We noticed a problem with your medical account. If you do not confirm your login today, your care may be delayed. Please click this **link** and enter your password right away. Thank you, Main Street Clinic Health Team

Figure 6-2: First Way Health

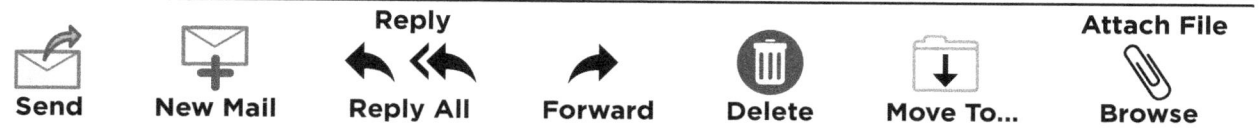

Email Folders	From:	First Way Health
Inbox Drafts Sent Deleted Items Junk Email Contacts	Subject:	Reminder: Your Appointment on October 19
	Message:	Hello, Leslie, This is a reminder of your appointment with Dr. Wyatt on Monday, October 19 at 9:00 a.m. at First Way Health. Please bring your insurance card and arrive 15 minutes early. Thank you, Your Care Team at First Way Health

Knowing how to spot a scam email, text or phone call is like checking if a stranger at your door is really who they say they are before letting them in. If something feels off, don't answer the door and certainly don't invite them in. In the case of a **phishing scam** like a fake email, don't take the bait. Stay alert and don't click on suspicious links or share personal information.

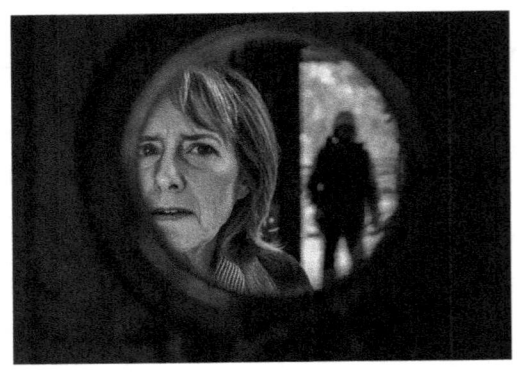

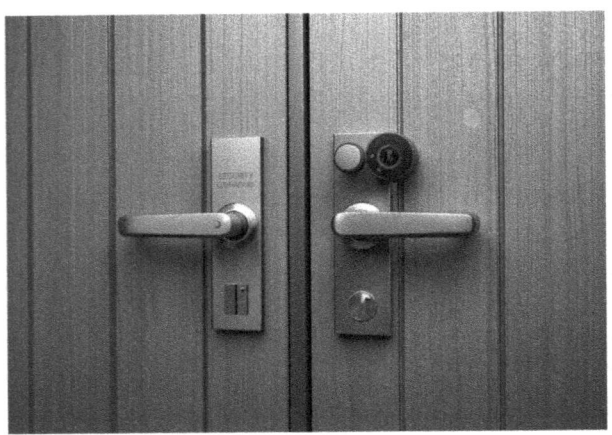

Using a strong password is like putting a strong lock on your front door. If your lock is weak, anyone can walk in. A good password keeps out intruders. Best practices for a strong password include using a mix of capital and lowercase letters, numbers, and symbols (like @ or !). You should also avoid passwords that include your name, birthday, guessable words, or simple number patterns like "1234."

Two-Factor Authentication

You should also turn on two-factor authentication, or 2FA. **Two-factor authentication** adds an extra step when you are logging in to an online account. In most instances, a code is sent to your phone or email to make sure it's really you. You must then enter this code when asked and submit it before gaining access to your account. If the code you enter is incorrect, you may need to repeat the process.

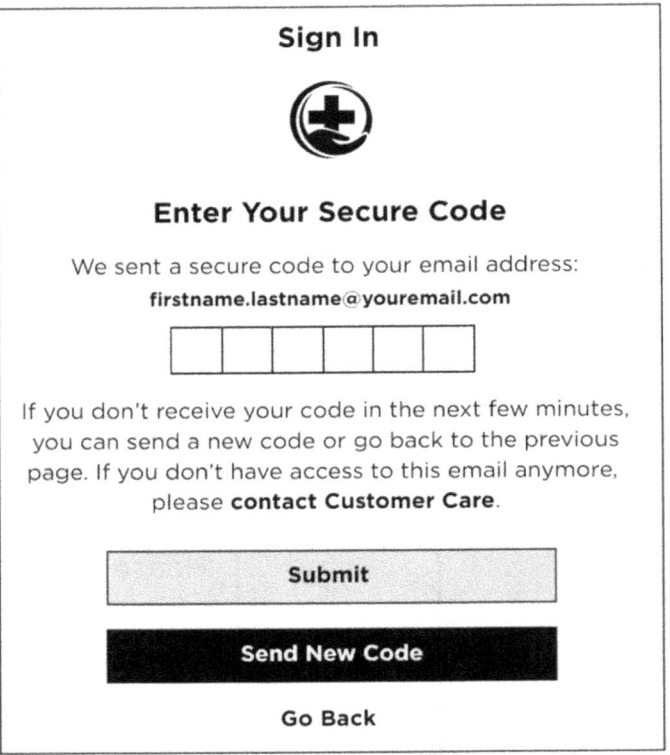

Figure 6-3: Two-Factor Authentication

It's also important to protect personal devices and accounts. Just like you wouldn't leave your wallet on a park bench, don't leave your phone or computer unlocked or share your login details. Keep them safe so no one else can use them to get your health information.

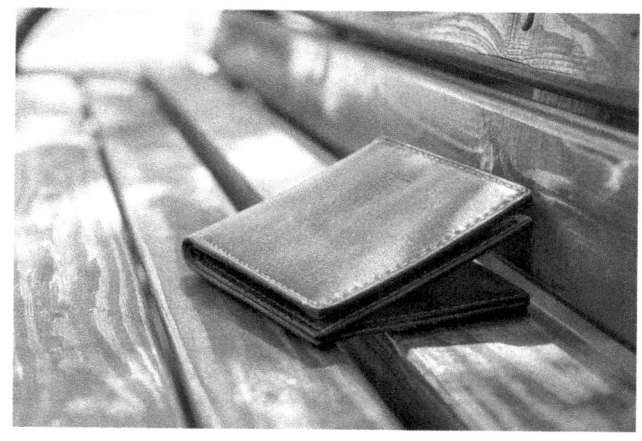

Finally, when using AI for fact-finding, be sure to double-check the output with a trusted doctor, nurse, or health professional before making decisions. Keep in mind that you are responsible for protecting your privacy by not sharing personal details like your full name, address, Social Security number, or medical ID numbers in your AI prompts.

The R.E.E.L.

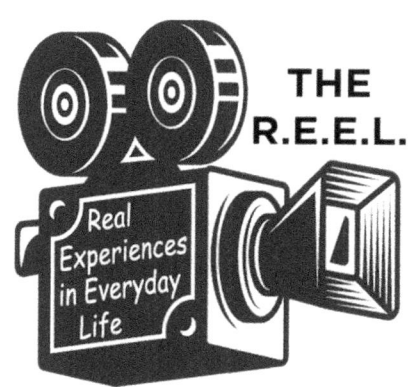

Healthcare Fraud

Healthcare fraud occurs when a company, clinic, or other provider tries to get money by lying about medical care, services, or supplies. During the COVID-19 pandemic, for example, some dishonest companies and clinics billed Medicare, Medicaid, and private insurance for COVID-19 PCR tests that patients never asked for or didn't need.[11,12]

Fight Back Against Healthcare Fraud

The following steps can help you put an end to healthcare fraud.

1. **Protect your insurance numbers.** Don't share your Medicare, Medicaid, or insurance ID with anyone except trusted doctors or clinics.
2. **Check your statements.** Look at your medical bills, Medicare/Medicaid summaries, or Explanations of Benefits (EOB) to make sure you only see services you really got.
3. **Speak up.** If you see charges for care or tests you didn't ask for or get, report it to your doctor's office, your insurance, or Medicare/Medicaid right away.

Activity #2

Directions: Read each question. Provide the **best** answer(s).

1. The table below contains twelve (12) potential passwords. Circle the **strong** passwords using the information you have learned about features of a good password.

987654321=	Password7	!25Dwq83Pfn	batman
bw?39P7dxp	flower	football	Trustno1
dragon	mZ26=f391B	princess	s94U$G593h

2. What does two-factor authentication (2FA) mean?

    A) Using two different doctors to confirm a **diagnosis,** which is the name for a health problem.

    B) Writing your password down in two places.

    C) Logging in twice to make sure your account is safe.

    D) Logging in with a password plus a second step, like a code.

3. Why is two-factor authentication safer than just a password?

    A) It makes logging in faster.

    B) It only works on mobile phones.

    C) It adds another layer of security if your password is stolen.

    D) It hides your password from your care team.

4. Judith is logging in to the online account provided by her health clinic. She receives a six digit code in her email and enters it. What should Judith do next? (Use **Figure 6-3** as a reference.)

    A) Click the "Send New Code" button.

    B) Click the "Submit" button.

    C) Go back to the previous page.

    D) Contact customer care.

5. Jorge is logging in to the online account provided by his health clinic. He receives a six digit code in his email, but he can't remember his email password. What should Jorge do next? (Use **Figure 6-3** as a reference.)

   A) Call his doctor and ask for the code over the phone.

   B) Keep guessing passwords until he gets into his email.

   C) Contact customer care.

   D) Ask a friend to log in to his email instead.

Keeping Care Safe

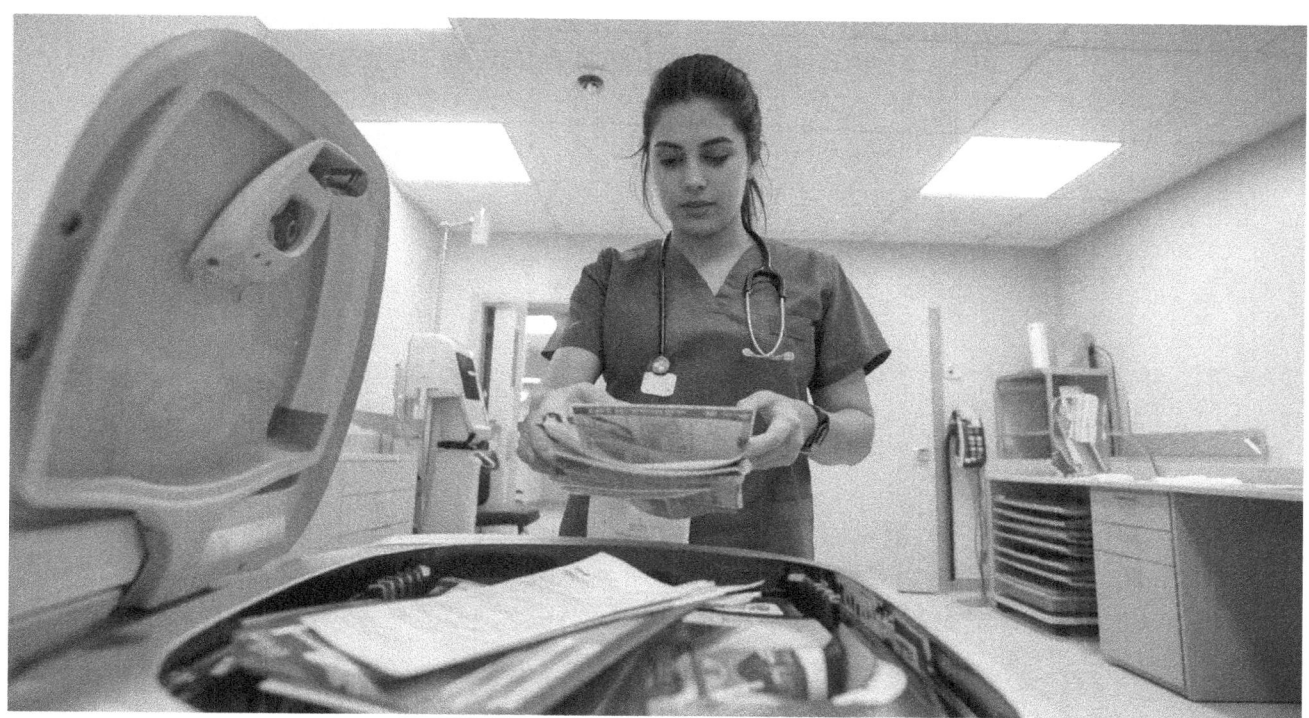

Doctors, nurses, and other care providers also have a responsibility to protect sensitive patient information. Not following HIPAA rules can lead to serious consequences like fines, required training or action plans, and even jail time.

According to Secureframe, a leading cybersecurity company, HIPAA violations can happen both by mistake and on purpose. Here are some common examples shared by Secureframe and The HIPAA Journal.[13,14]

- Talking about a patient's condition in a public place where others can hear.
- Looking at a patient's record out of curiosity, without a work reason.

- Sending protected health information (PHI) to a personal email account to finish work at home.
- Leaving a laptop with PHI unlocked on a desk when stepping away.
- Posting a photo on social media that shows a hospital room with patient information visible.
- Throwing paper records with patient information in the trash instead of shredding them.

Staff often have issues with protecting sensitive health information because they may talk about patients in public areas, forget how easily private details can be overheard, or feel rushed and careless under pressure. Sometimes they don't realize that casual conversations or sharing too much information can break patient trust and violate privacy rules, even with good intentions.

If your private health information is being handled the wrong way, it's important to speak up. Speaking up protects you, builds trust, and helps keep care safe for everyone. You can also file a complaint with the Department of Health and Human Services Office for Civil Rights (OCR) or ask your state's attorney general for help.

Activity #3

Directions: Read each scenario. Then, write what should have been done differently, if anything, to keep the patient's information safe and private, and avoid a HIPAA violation.

1. **Sharing Without Permission.** A surgery clinic gave a patient's private health information to a research group without asking the patient first or getting approval from a review board.

   _____

   _____

2. **Withholding Records.** A doctor's office refused to give a patient their medical records because the patient still owed money.

   _____

   _____

3. **Calling a Patient's Name.** A nurse calls out, "Miguel Lopez?" in the waiting room to bring him back for his appointment.

_____

_____

4. **Unnecessary Sharing.** A hospital emailed an Operating Room schedule to staff that included details about an employee's surgery, which their supervisor (not part of the treatment team) could see.

_____

_____

5. **Labels That Expose.** A dental office put a red sticker that said "No COVID Vaccine" on some patient charts, where anyone could see it.

_____

_____

6. **Family Member at the Visit.** A patient brings her husband into the exam room. The doctor talks about her diagnosis with both of them present.

_____

_____

7. **No Privacy Notice.** A mental health center did not give a father and his daughter (the patient) a written notice explaining how the daughter's health information would be used before her evaluation.

_____

_____

_____

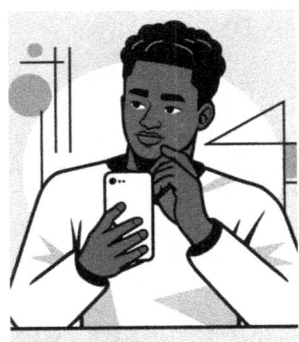

Show What You Know!

Congratulations on completing the lesson. You've made great progress. Enter your site code and the information below to answer a few quick questions about what you learned.

| Lesson Six | Checkpoint Number: **12** |

Key Terms

Care Operations	The behind-the-scenes activities that clinics and hospitals do to make patient care safe, organized, and better.
Diagnosis	The name for a health problem.
Healthcare Fraud	A dishonest act that occurs when a company, clinic, or other provider tries to get money by lying about medical care, services, or supplies.
HIPAA	Short for the Health Insurance Portability and Accountability Act, which is a law that protects personal health information and makes sure doctors, nurses, and clinics keep it private and secure.
Notice of Privacy Practices (NPP)	A written notice that explains how your health information may be shared.
Orthodontist	A type of dentist who is trained to fix crooked teeth and jaws, often by using braces or clear aligners.
Phishing Scam	A fake email, text, or message that looks real, but is designed to trick you into giving away personal information, like a password or bank account number.
Security Awareness Training	An educational practice that teaches how to spot online threats, protect your accounts, and keep sensitive information safe.
Two-Factor Authentication	An extra step when logging in that asks for a code, fingerprint, or other proof of identity along with your password.

LESSON SEVEN: Working with Your Care Team

Introduction

Objectives – After completing this lesson, you will be able to:
- Explain how patients, families, staff, and community can work together to improve health
- Point out the good results that come from partnering
- Practice filling out a survey about your own care experience
- Show how everyone in the circle of care can do their part to keep care safe and effective
- Understand why the patient's voice matters for stronger teamwork and to prevent missed chances

Key Terms

- Allergist
- Circle of Care
- Dermatologist
- Early Intervention

- Feedback
- Mites
- Shared Responsibility
- Topical Cream

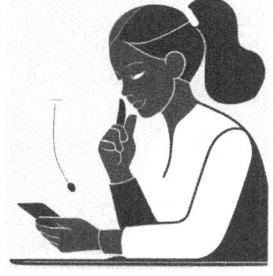

Let's Get Started!

Your voice matters. Enter your site code and the information below to share what you already know and what you hope to learn about working with your care team.

Lesson Seven	Checkpoint Number: **13**

Teaming Up for Positive Outcomes

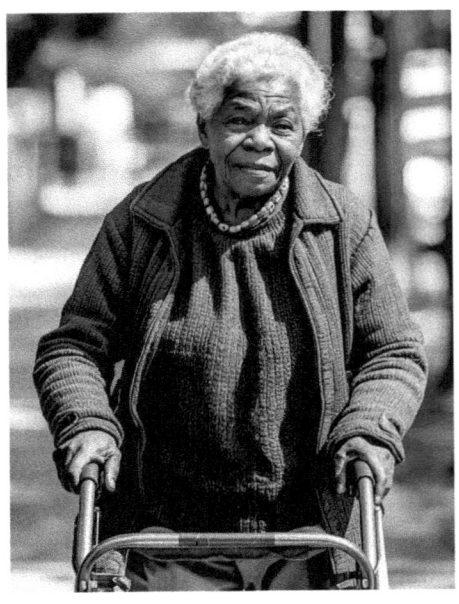

Good health care works best when patients and care teams partner together and share responsibility. By working as a team — asking questions, giving feedback, and using digital tools — everyone can help make care safer, easier, and more effective.

The circle of care introduced in Lesson One shows that good health care takes a team. Your circle of care is the support system that connects you with people, places, meaningful technology, and your health information. It includes people, places, and tools that work together to keep you healthy.

When someone has surgery, for example, healing is not something they do alone. Doctors, nurses, pharmacies, family, and digital tools like health apps and AI all play a part in recovery. The following hip surgery example shows how the circle of care works together to help the patient (Mrs. Lovejoy) heal and stay safe.

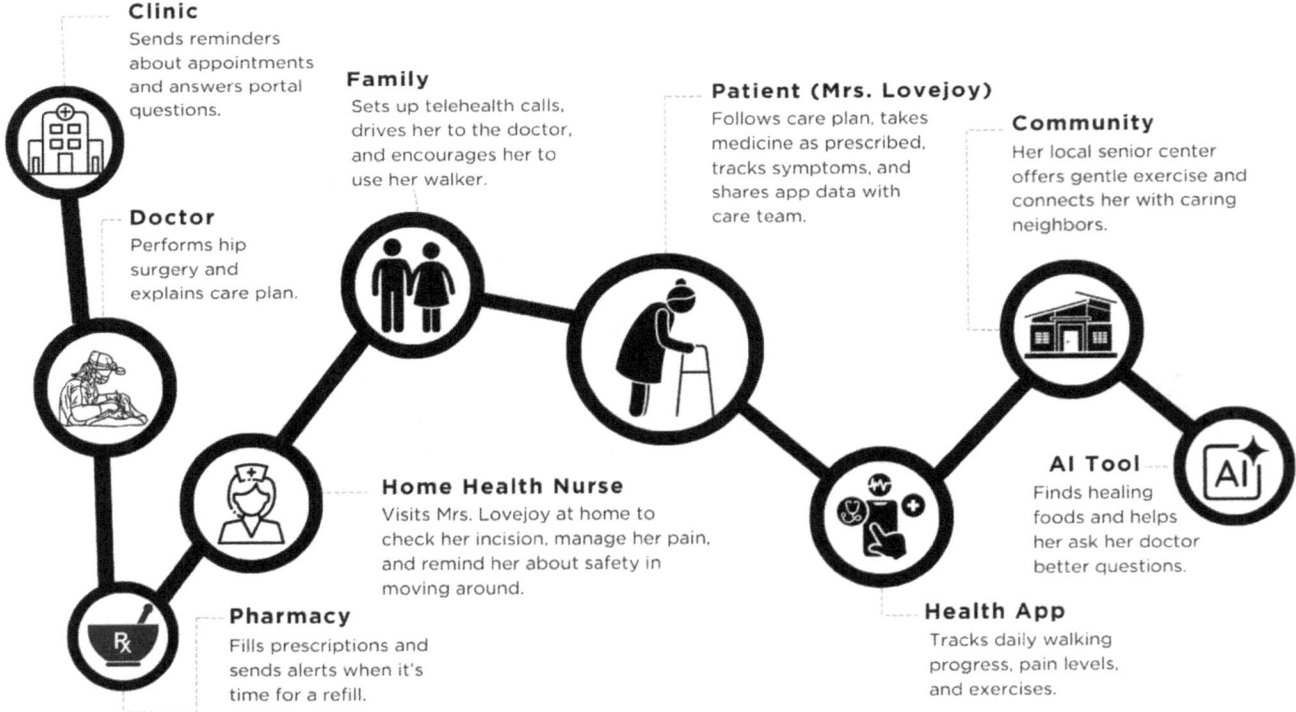

Figure 7-1: Recovery After Hip Surgery

Partnering means patients, care teams, and digital health tools each do their part. When that happens, care is safer, problems are caught earlier, medicines work better, and support goes beyond the clinic or hospital. By coordinating, working together, and holding each other accountable, patients, family, and staff can reach better outcomes — like keeping up with medicines, staying on track with screenings, catching problems sooner (**early intervention**), and making sure social needs are met.

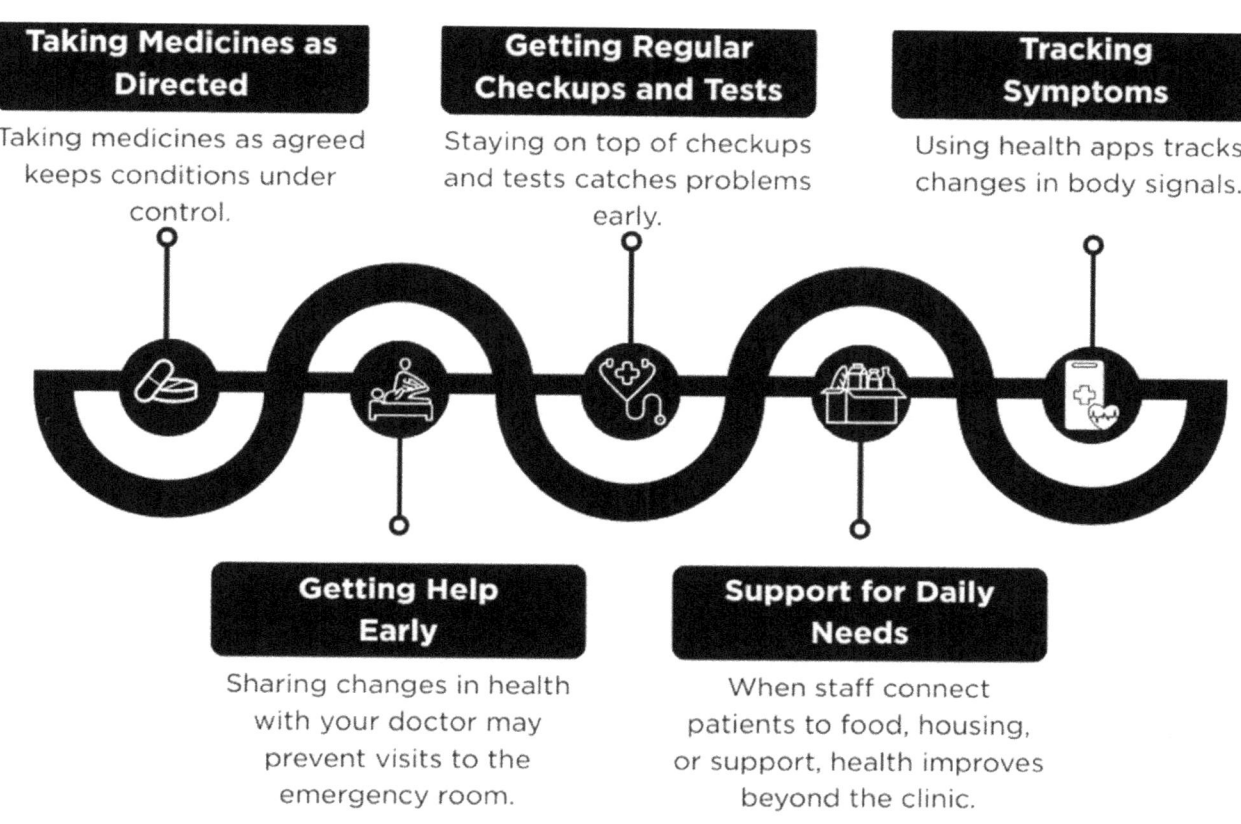

Figure 7-2: Positive Outcomes of Partnering

Activity #1

Directions: Read each scenario. Refer to **Figure 7-2** to describe the positive outcome.

1. Tammy notices swelling in her ankles and messages her doctor through the patient portal. Her care team adjusts her medicine right away, and she avoids kidney failure.

   _____

   _____

2. Paul goes to his yearly checkup and gets a cancer screening. The test finds a small problem early, and it is treated before it gets worse.

   _____

   _____

3. Mr. Grant takes his blood pressure medicine every day as prescribed. At his next checkup, his blood pressure is under control, and he no longer feels dizzy.

   _____

   _____

4. Ms. Alvarez struggles to get healthy food because she doesn't drive. Her clinic connects her with a local food delivery program. With better meals and exercise, her diabetes is under control.

   _____

   _____

5. Rosa uses a health app to track her blood sugar and notice which foods make it go up or down. By changing what she eats and sharing the numbers with her nurse, her blood sugar improves and she moves from diabetic to pre-diabetic.

   _____

   _____

Feedback to Improve Care

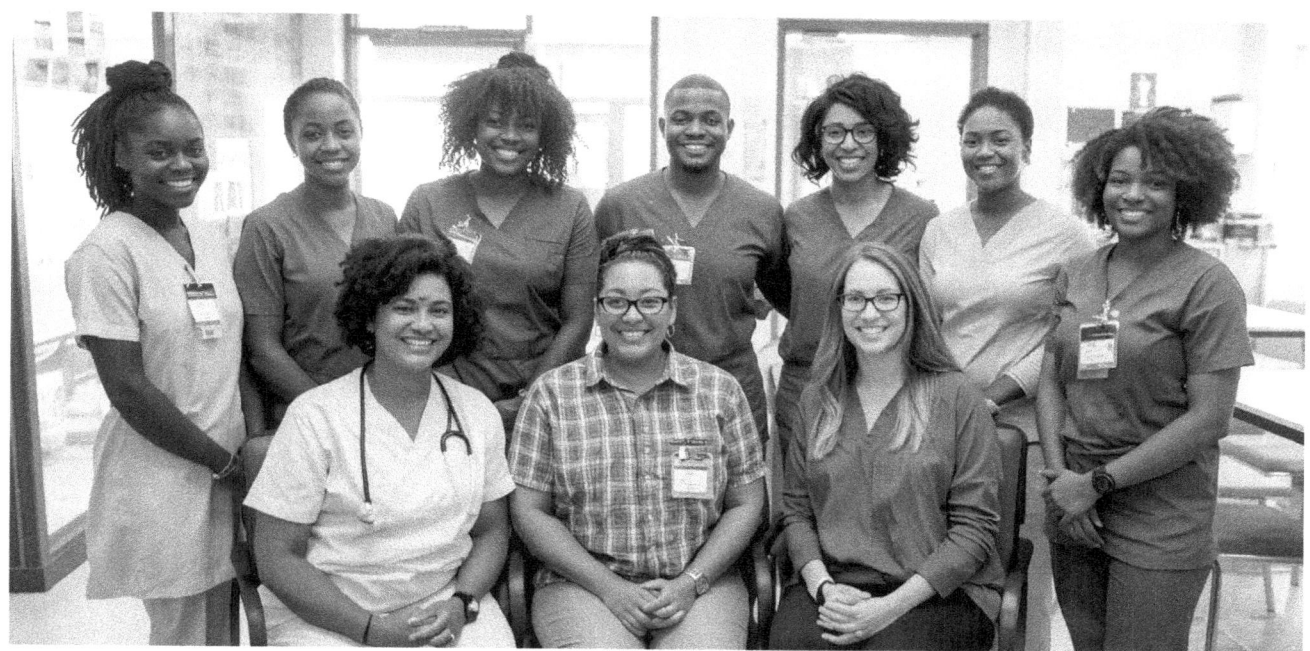

Good health care takes teamwork. Patients, families, doctors, nurses, and community helpers all play a role in the circle of care. By giving and receiving **feedback**, each person helps the team understand what's working, what needs to change, and how to keep care safe and effective.

Feedback can come from patient surveys, care team input, and community support. Data and AI are also helpful because they show big-picture trends, but it is people working together every day that really improves care and health outcomes.

- **Patient Feedback (surveys, direct input):** Patients share their experiences, and the care team uses it to adjust and improve.
- **Care Team Feedback (peer-to-peer):** Doctors, nurses, medical assistants,

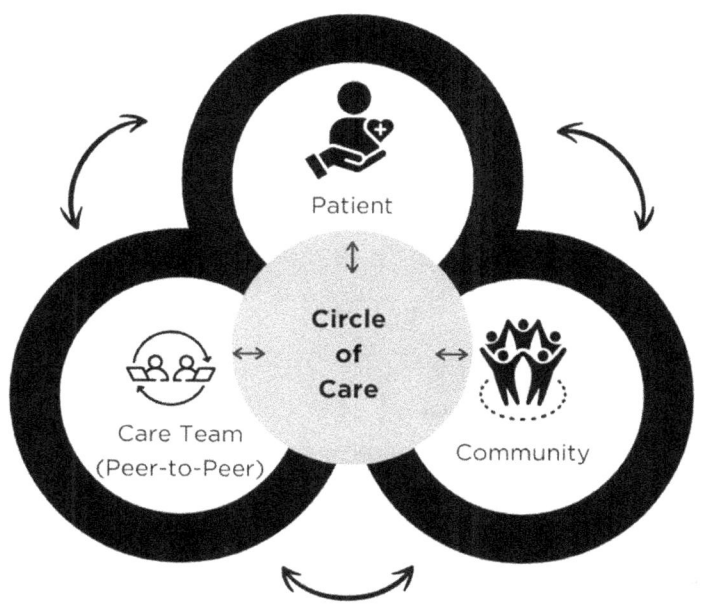

Figure 7-3: Human Feedback That Strengthens Partnership

community health workers, and other frontline staff give feedback to each other so handoffs, communication, and digital tools work smoothly.

- **Community Feedback:** When outside partners (like food programs or senior centers) report back on whether patients received help, it extends the partnership beyond the clinic and shows how care connects to social needs.

Activity #2

Practice Survey: How Was Your Care Experience?

Directions – Part A: Think back to a recent visit with a doctor, nurse, or health worker — either in person or by phone/video. This survey helps you think about what worked well and where things could improve. Circle the answer that best matches your experience. If a question doesn't apply to your situation (for example, you don't take medicine), record 2 points so your total stays consistent.

1. How well did your provider listen to you?
    - (3) They really listened and gave me time to speak
    - (2) They listened some of the time
    - (1) They seemed rushed or distracted

2. How clearly did they explain your health or treatment?
    - (3) Very clear — I understood everything
    - (2) Somewhat clear — I had a few questions
    - (1) Not clear — I was confused or unsure

3. Did you feel respected by the provider and staff?
    - (3) Yes, completely
    - (2) Kind of — some things could have been better
    - (1) No, I didn't feel respected

4. Did you have a chance to ask questions?
    - (3) Yes — and they answered clearly
    - (2) I asked, but the answers weren't very helpful
    - (1) I didn't feel like I could ask questions

5. Were you told what to do after your visit (for example, take medicine, schedule another visit, or check your blood pressure)?
    - (3) Yes, everything was explained clearly
    - (2) Some of it — I had to figure out the rest
    - (1) No, I left confused

6. How easy was it to schedule your appointment?
    - (3) Very easy — I had no problems
    - (2) It took some effort
    - (1) It was hard or confusing

7. Did your provider include you in decisions about your care?
    - (3) Yes — I helped make the decisions
    - (2) Somewhat — I was told the options
    - (1) No — decisions were made without asking me

8. Did anyone ask about things that make it hard for you to stay healthy? (e.g., food, housing, transportation, caregiving)
    - (3) Yes — they asked and listened
    - (2) Yes — but they didn't follow up
    - (1) No — no one asked

9. Did you understand your medicine instructions (if any)?
    - (3) Yes — I knew what to take and why
    - (2) Sort of — I had to guess
    - (1) No — it was confusing or unclear

10. Did your provider explain the benefits and risks of your treatment or medicine in a way you could understand?
    - (3) Yes — I understood the benefits and risks
    - (2) Somewhat — I still had questions
    - (1) No — the risks and side effects were unclear

11. Did you feel you had a real choice to accept or refuse the treatment or medicine after it was explained to you?
    - (3) Yes, I felt fully informed and had a choice
    - (2) Somewhat, but I wasn't sure
    - (1) No, I didn't feel I had a choice

12. Did your provider or care team make good use of digital tools (like patient portals, telehealth, or health apps) to support your care?

    (3) Yes, the tools were easy to use and helpful

    (2) Somewhat, the tools were used but could be better

    (1) No, the tools were not used or not helpful

Survey Results

Directions – Part B (Your Score): Add your numbers from each question.

My Total: _____ / 36

Total Points	What It Means
31-36	Excellent care experience. You felt heard, informed, and part of the team.
25-30	Good care experience, but there may be small areas that could be better.
19-24	Fair care experience. Some important things were missing or unclear.
12-18	Poor care experience. Many areas need improvement.

Partnering Across Digital Health Skills

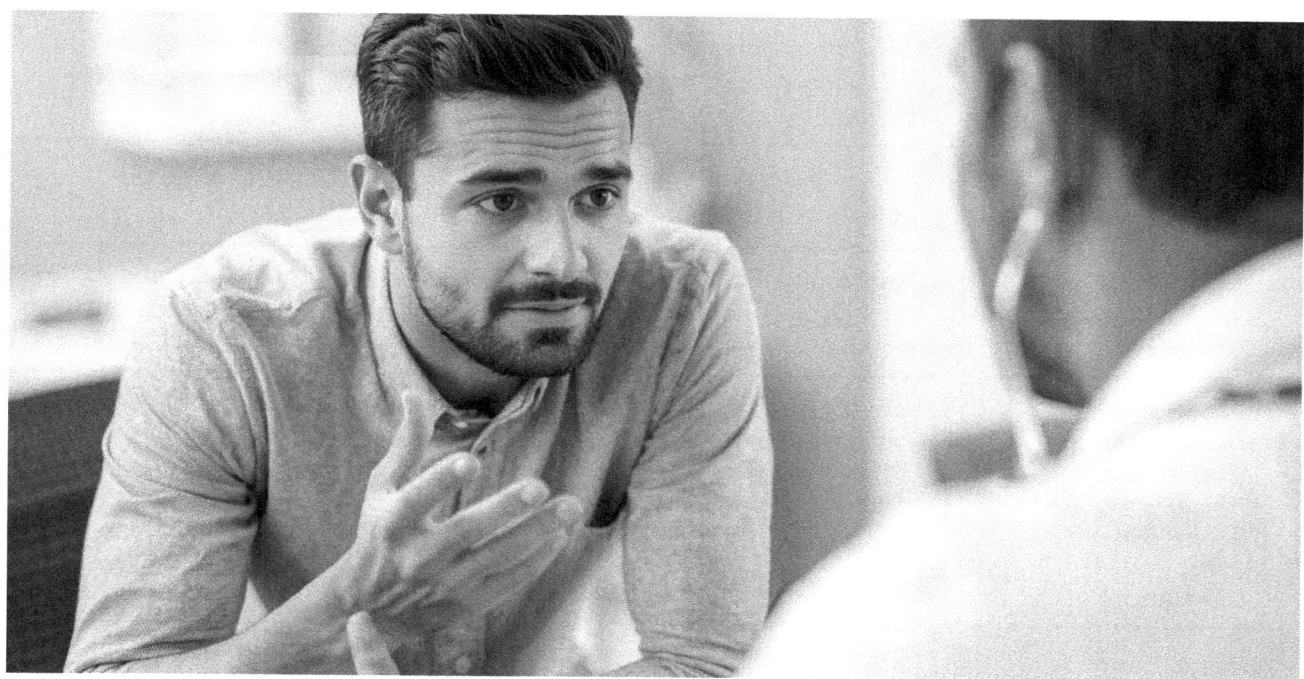

Each skill covered in this workbook helps make care smoother, safer, and less stressful. From using patient portals and preparing for telehealth visits to choosing the right place of care or protecting sensitive health data, patients and staff have a role to play. Asking questions, speaking up, and holding everyone accountable is a shared responsibility to ensure quality care for self and others. **Shared responsibility** means all circle of care participants do their part to keep care safe and effective.

The following table summarizes how partnering across every digital health skill leads to better outcomes and strengthens trust.

Lesson Topic	Shared Responsibility
Lesson One — Identifying Your Circle of Care	Patient and staff identify the patient's support system and the role each participant plays, including technology.
Lesson One — Choosing the Right Place of Care	Patient and staff work together to decide if care should be in-person, by video, or through an e-visit.
Lesson Two — Online Patient Portals	Patients log in to check their test results, see reminders for checkups and screenings, and send messages to their care team. Staff respond quickly to keep communication clear.

Lesson Topic	Shared Responsibility
Lesson Three — Telehealth Visits	Patient becomes comfortable booking an appointment online and using AI to prepare for a video visit, while staff make sure the technology and visit go smoothly.
Lesson Four — Using Mobile Health Apps	Patient tracks habits like food, steps, or sugar intake, and staff review this information to support daily health goals.
Lesson Four — Remote Patient Monitoring	Devices like blood pressure cuffs or wearables track the patient's body signals and send updates to the clinic, helping staff catch problems early.
Lesson Five — Trusting Health Information	Patients learn to spot propaganda and cognitive bias. Both patients and staff use tools like the CLEAR Head Approach to sort facts from misinformation and make smart choices with a calm, clear mind.
Lesson Six — Protecting Health Information	Patients and staff keep data safe by using strong passwords, two-factor authentication, and avoiding scams.
Lesson Seven — Working as a Team	Patients, staff, and community give and receive feedback to keep the circle of care strong and help everyone stay accountable.

By working together and building confidence in the use of digital health skills, patients and staff can reach better outcomes — from taking medicines on time to getting screenings and finding help with daily needs. Using AI wisely can also support this teamwork by helping explain information, prepare questions, and guide choices, while still checking with trusted professionals.

The R.E.E.L.

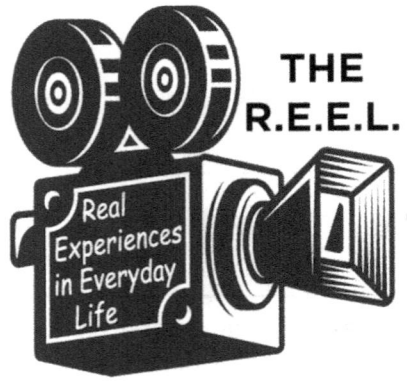

Speaking Up

The following story is about an 81-year-old woman who followed her doctor's orders and used AI to learn more about her health, but was afraid to speak up.

Directions: Read each step in Debbie's story. At each step, decide if it shows Strong Partnership or a Missed Opportunity. Circle your choice and answer the reflection questions that follow.

Step 1 – First Visit

Debbie, age 81, develops a skin rash she's never had before. She tells her doctor, who sends her to an **allergist** (a doctor who tests and treats people for allergies, like reactions to food, pollen, or medicine). The allergy tests come back negative.

    Strong Partnership   Missed Opportunity

Step 2 – Using AI

Debbie describes her symptoms to an AI tool. The AI suggests the correct diagnosis and treatment: an oral medicine plus a **topical cream** (a medicine you rub on your skin to treat a problem in that area). Debbie's daughter does similar research and encourages her to ask the doctor about the oral medicine.

    Strong Partnership   Missed Opportunity

Step 3 – Dermatologist Visit

Debbie's doctor refers her to a **dermatologist** (a doctor who treats problems with the skin, hair, and nails). The dermatologist prescribes only the cream. Debbie does not mention what the AI suggested, and her daughter confirmed, about the oral medicine.

    Strong Partnership   Missed Opportunity

Step 4 – Follow-Up

At her follow-up visit, Debbie tells the dermatologist the rash is better but she still has itching. The dermatologist says she's fine and needs no more treatment.

    Strong Partnership   Missed Opportunity

Step 5 – Outcome

Two weeks later, the rash comes back. Debbie realizes the **mites** (tiny bugs that can lay eggs under the skin and cause itching and rashes) are still in her system. She wishes she had spoken up about what the AI suggested.

    Strong Partnership   Missed Opportunity

Reflection Questions:

1. What could have changed if Debbie had shared the AI's suggestion with her dermatologist?

_____

_____

2. Why is it important for patients to speak up, even if they think the doctor knows more?

_____

_____

3. How can staff encourage patients like Debbie to share what they learn from digital tools?

_____

_____

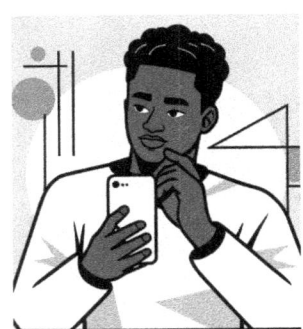

Show What You Know!

Congratulations on completing the lesson. You've made great progress. Enter your site code and the information below to answer a few quick questions about what you learned.

| Lesson Seven | Checkpoint Number: **14** |

Key Terms

Allergist	A doctor who tests and treats people for allergies, like reactions to food, pollen, or medicine.
Circle of Care	A support system that connects you with people, places, meaningful technology, and your health information.
Dermatologist	A doctor who treats problems with the skin, hair, and nails.
Early Intervention	Getting help at the first sign of a problem so it doesn't turn into an emergency.
Feedback	Information you give or receive to show what is working well and what needs to improve.
Mites	Tiny bugs that can lay eggs under the skin and cause itching and rashes.

Shared Responsibility When patients, families, and health teams all do their part to keep care safe and effective.

Topical Cream A medicine you rub on your skin to treat a problem in that area.

Acknowledgments

This project would not have been possible without the dedication of educators and trainers who put the workbook into practice and tested the checkpoint system with their learners. Special thanks to **Cathy Elizondo** (Workforce Instructional Specialist, Central Arizona College), **Laurel Dennis** (Library Assistant, Placentia Library District), and **Abigail Causey** (Digital Navigator, National Church Residences) for their commitment to helping learners build skills and for providing valuable feedback on the usefulness of the digital health content and the checkpoint data.

We are also grateful to **New Readers Press** for helping recruit pilot sites, and to **First Baptist Church** (Raleigh, NC) and **Durham County Public Library** for hosting pilot cohorts. Their support and participation helped shape the system that now connects digital health training with measurable outcomes.

About the Author

ANGELA HARRIS is the creator of the Tech-for-Care Advocate™ system and author of the *One Click at a Time* digital skills series, used by educators and trainers in more than 40 states and Canada. A leader in digital inclusion and workforce development, she combines instructional design, professional training, and the integration of AI in workflows to equip organizations with tools that improve impact and accountability. Her workbooks and training programs connect digital skills to measurable outcomes, helping staff and learners build confidence in real-world settings while giving organizations clear ways to track and reward the impact of training. Angela frequently speaks at national conferences on adult and continuing education, sharing insights on digital skill-building, multi-stakeholder collaboration, and the future of workforce training.

ENDNOTES

1. Abd-Alrazaq, A. A., Bewick, B. M., Farragher, T., & Gardner, P. (2019). Factors that affect the use of electronic personal health records among patients: A systematic review. *International Journal of Medical Informatics*, 126, 164–175. https://www.sciencedirect.com/science/article/abs/pii/S1386505618312255?via%3Dihub.

2. Avera Health. (2019, May 22). *How much sugar is in your drink?* [Video]. YouTube. https://www.youtube.com/watch?v=i6NBIqLHp2o.

3. Chai, C. (2012, June 8). *How many spoonfuls of sugar are in your drink?* Global News. https://globalnews.ca/news/254160/how-many-spoonfuls-of-sugar-are-in-your-drink/.

4. Cleveland Clinic. (2023, February 21). *What Is a Normal Body Temperature?* Cleveland Clinic. https://health.clevelandclinic.org/body-temperature-what-is-and-isnt-normal.

5. American Heart Association. (2025, August 14). *Understanding blood pressure readings.* https://www.heart.org/en/health-topics/high-blood-pressure/understanding-blood-pressure-readings.

6. American Diabetes Association. (n.d.). *Understanding diabetes diagnosis.* Retrieved from https://diabetes.org/about-diabetes/diagnosis.

7. Mayo Clinic. (2022, October 8). *What's a normal resting heart rate?* Mayo Clinic. https://www.mayoclinic.org/healthy-lifestyle/fitness/expert-answers/heart-rate/faq-20057979.

8. Mayo Clinic Staff. (2023, March 24). *Low blood oxygen (hypoxemia) – definition.* Mayo Clinic. https://www.mayoclinic.org/symptoms/hypoxemia/basics/definition/sym-20050930.

9. CPR Care. (2025, August 28). *Normal respiratory rate in adults: What you need to know.* CPRCare. https://cprcare.com/blog/normal-respiratory-rate-for-adults/.

10. AAMC. (2024, June 27). *Microplastics are inside us all. What does that mean for our health?* AAMC. https://www.aamc.org/news/microplastics-are-inside-us-all-what-does-mean-our-health.

11. Small, B. (2023, June 8). *Medicare fraud prevention: What's on your statement?* Federal Trade Commission. https://consumer.ftc.gov/consumer-alerts/2023/06/medicare-fraud-prevention-whats-your-statement.

12. Smith, D. J., Brater, R. A., Dearington, M. F., Patel, N., Stemple, H. M., & Foreman, R. W. (2024, June 14). *Chicago laboratory owner charged with defrauding Medicare in $60 million COVID-19 test kit scheme.* ArentFox Schiff. https://www.afslaw.com/perspectives/investigations-blog/chicago-laboratory-owner-charged-defrauding-medicare-60-million.

13. HIPAA Journal. (2025). *What is a HIPAA violation?* HIPAA Journal. https://www.hipaajournal.com/what-is-a-hipaa-violation/.

14. Secureframe. (2025, August 18). *HIPAA violation examples in 2025: 20 common violations with real-world enforcement cases.* Secureframe. https://secureframe.com/hub/hipaa/violations.

Digital Health: One Click at a Time

ANSWER KEYS

ANSWERS — LESSON ONE: What is Digital Health?

The R.E.E.L.

Because healthy food, safe places to live, reliable transportation, and steady work are basic needs that affect a person's health, the circle of care is expanding to include a person's social environment.

Directions: Use the information in the passage and knowledge about your community to answer each question.

1. Who is in your circle of care?

    Answers will vary.

2. Dana lives in another part of the country and is caring for her elderly mom who lives in **your community**. What resources are available to provide a hot meal or healthy food for Dana's mom who stays at home and is recovering from an illness?

    Answers will vary.

3. When Dana's mom recovers and becomes active again, what resources are available in **your community** to ensure that she maintains her wellbeing and social connections?

    Answers will vary.

Activity #1

Directions: It's time to check your understanding of digital health. Read each question. Circle the **best** answer.

1. When thinking about how people use technology for care, which answer best describes the **circle of care**?

    A) An online meeting place where doctors go to learn new skills.

    (B) A team of people using digital tools to work together and give a person the care they need.

    C) The care team members shown in an individual's patient portal.

2. Susan's doctor has been treating her acne with a prescription medication. Susan just completed her last refill and now needs to request more of the same medication. Which of these places of care is the best choice for Susan?

    A) Video call   B) In-person visit   **(C)** E-Visit

3. Victoria has received X-ray results regarding the arthritis in her right knee. She desires a follow-up visit with her doctor. Which of these places of care is the best choice for her follow-up visit?

    A) In-person visit   B) E-Visit   **(C) Video call**

Explanation: Victoria can have a video call with her doctor to talk about her X-ray results. The doctor can explain what the X-ray shows and tell her what to do next. Given that this is a follow-up visit, Victoria doesn't need to go into the office because the doctor already saw her and knows about her condition.

4. Larry twists his ankle during basketball practice and his coach tells him that it can be treated with rest, ice, compression, and elevation, also known as RICE. The coach further explains that RICE is a simple first-aid method used to treat sudden injuries like sprains, pulled muscles, and bruises. Which of these places of care is the best, immediate choice to take care of Larry?

    (A) Rest at home
    B) Urgent care
    C) Video call

5. **True** or **False**. Write **T** for True or **F** for False next to the statements below.

    __F__   A) Digital health makes it less likely to be confused by unfamiliar health words and tools.

Explanation: This statement is false. Digital health terms and tools can be hard to understand without help.

    __T__   B) Carter is wearing a ring that tracks his body temperature and sleep patterns. He is most likely wearing a smart ring, which is a type of wearable device.

Explanation: This statement is true. Carter's ring is worn on the finger and connected to the internet, tracking various health data. These features describe a wearable device.

6. Now that you have seen some examples of wearable devices in the lesson, let's see if you can spot them on your own. Below are four pictures. Look at each one and identify the type of wearable device.

    A) _Smart Watch_
    B) _Heart Rate Monitor_
    C) _Virtual Reality (VR) Headset or Goggles_
    D) _Continuous Glucose Monitor_

Activity #2

Directions: Read each question and provide the **best** answer.

1. Donald is about to have two extra teeth removed by his dentist. Before the procedure, his dentist asks which pharmacy to send a prescription for pain medicine. After his appointment, Donald plans to stop by his local grocery store to buy soft foods that are easy to chew. He likes how convenient the grocery store is and knows the pharmacy there has great service. Which pharmacy is Donald most likely to choose for his prescription?

    A) Amazon Pharmacy (online)
    B) Kroger Pharmacy (retail)
    C) Express Scripts (mail-order)

2. Alice likes that her insurance covers a 90-day supply of insulin and that it can be delivered to her home for free. Because her feet are often swollen and it's hard for her to get around, which pharmacy is she most likely to choose for her long-term medicine?

    A) Jackson's Neighborhood Pharmacy
    B) Express Scripts
    C) Kroger Pharmacy

3. Jack values having a face-to-face relationship with the medical professionals in his circle of care. He thinks it's best to get all his prescriptions from the same pharmacy chain. Today, Jack is leaving work early to pick up his arthritis medicine. Which pharmacy is he most likely going to after work?

    A) Jackson's Neighborhood Pharmacy
    B) Amazon Pharmacy
    C) Walgreens

4. Tabitha is reviewing a prescription bottle, which instructs her to take 1 tablet each day for 60 days. How many tablets will Tabitha take in 60 days?

    A) 30 tablets
    B) 60 tablets
    C) 120 tablets
    D) 240 tablets

5. What does it mean that Tabitha has 4 refills?

   It means after she finishes her first 60-day supply, she can get four more 60-day supplies of the same medicine without needing a new prescription.

   Answers will vary.

6. How can Tabitha use her patient portal to manage her prescription?

   Tabitha can log in to her patient portal to see her prescription details, request a refill, or message her doctor if she has questions about the medicine.

   Answers will vary.

7. What is one way Tabitha's pharmacy might use technology to help her remember to take her medicine?

   The pharmacy might send text message reminders or let Tabitha use a mobile app that sends alerts when it's time to take her pill or refill her prescription.

   Answers will vary.

8. Which of the following is not likely to be found in a person's electronic health record (EHR)?
   - A) Date of birth
   - **B) Insurance policy number**
   - C) Unshared home remedies
   - D) Lab results

9. Based on the information in the passage, explain **telehealth** in your own words.

   Telehealth is healthcare assistance without leaving home; obtaining care using technology; online visits with your doctor.

   Answers will vary.

Activity #3

Directions: Peter, Maria, Jorge, Ivan, and Cathy want a mobile app to manage their health. Review each app below. Then, use the comments made by each individual to select the mobile health app that will help them achieve their goals.

1 2 3 4 5

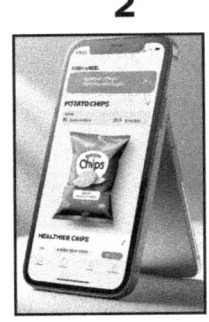 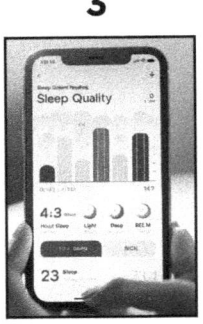 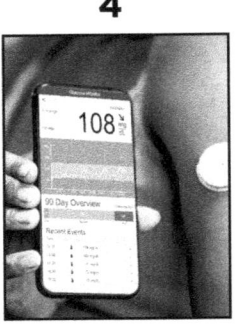 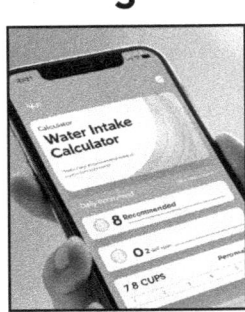

Patient	Comments	Best App (Write the Number)
Peter	"I need a way to see how my blood sugar changes during the day. I have type 2 diabetes and want to eat better to stay healthy."	4
Maria	"My doctor told me I'm not drinking enough water. I need a reminder to help me drink the right amount each day based on my weight and daily activity."	5
Jorge	"I want a tool that helps me take better care of my high blood pressure. I also want to learn what makes it go up or down."	1
Ivan	"I don't sleep well. I want to track my sleep so I can learn how to improve my rest and make better choices."	3
Cathy	"I love salty snacks! I'd like a tool I can use while shopping to scan foods and help me pick healthier options."	2

Activity #4

Directions: Sofia is committed to making better health choices and is experimenting with AI to achieve this goal. You are invited to come along for the journey and learn with Sofia. Read each question and provide the **best** answer.

1. Sofia takes a picture of her dinner before eating the meal and shares a photo (in color) of the food on her plate with her favorite AI tool. She asks the AI to tell her about this meal.

    True or **False**. Write **T** for True or **F** for False next to the statements below.

    _____T_____ A) The AI tool is able to review the picture and identify every food on the plate.

    Explanation: This statement is true. The AI correctly identifies the meal as grilled salmon, roasted sweet potatoes, steamed kale, and white rice.

    _____T_____ B) When prompted, the AI is able to estimate the total calories of the entire meal.

    Explanation: This statement is true. The AI provides a calorie estimate for each individual item and the entire meal.

2. Sofia's AI tool provides an overall meal assessment. Which of the following is not part of the meal assessment?

    A) Heart-healthy
    B) Diabetes-friendly (with portion control)
    C) Unbalanced
    D) Great for recovery

    Explanation: The overall meal assessment includes feedback pointing to a well-balanced meal due to the inclusion of a protein, healthy fats, complex carbs, and plenty of vitamins and minerals.

3. Which one of Sofia's food items is most likely described as being "good for heart and brain health?"

    A) Roasted Sweet Potatoes
    B) Grilled Salmon
    C) Steamed Kale

    Explanation: According to the AI tool and available food data, the grilled salmon is considered good for heart and brain health due to its rich content of omega-3 fatty acids.

4. The AI tool identifies the following health benefits for one of Sofia's dinner items: good for eye health, digestion, and provides long-lasting energy. Which dinner item is most likely to have these benefits?
   - **(A) Roasted Sweet Potatoes**
   - B) Grilled Salmon
   - C) Steamed Kale

5. Based on the information that Sofia is receiving about her dinner from AI, how could you adopt this practice to make better decisions about what you eat over time?

   You can take pictures of your meals and use an AI tool to learn what's in your food – like calories and nutrition. You can also track what you eat and combine it with other health data, such as weight or blood pressure, to see how your meals affect your health. Over time, this can help you make smarter choices and build healthier habits.

   Answers will vary.

Activity #5

Directions: Read each question. Use the summary lab results above to provide the **best** answer.

1. Which test checks whether Sofia is getting enough **hydration**, or water?
   - A) Glucose
   - **(B) BUN**
   - C) Creatinine

2. Which test measures the amount of a simple sugar in the blood?
   - **(A) Glucose**
   - B) BUN
   - C) Creatinine

3. **True** or **False.** Write **T** for True or **F** for False next to the statements below.

   ___T___   A) Sofia's lab results communicate a positive update.

   Explanation: This statement is true. Sofia's blood sugar, hydration, and kidney function currently look good. Her results are either steady or improving compared to her last test.

3. **True** or **False.** Write **T** for True or **F** for False next to the statements below.

   __T__   B) If Sofia has concerns about the accuracy of her summary results, she can ask the AI to share its sources.

   Explanation: This statement is true. Sofia can ask the AI to share the source of its data. She can also ask her doctor or look at trusted medical websites like Mayo Clinic or MedlinePlus to double-check what the numbers mean.

4. What is an effective prompt, or question, Sofia can ask to learn how her diet may affect these lab results?

   Can you please explain how these labs relate to what I eat, and what foods I should choose or avoid?.

   Answers will vary.

ANSWERS — LESSON TWO: Online Patient Portals

The R.E.E.L.

Directions: Kira wants to log in to her patient portal. She remembers her username, but can't remember her password. What should she do? Use the Patient Portal Login Page image to assist you.

Kira should click the "Forgot Password" link on the login page. She will be asked to answer a few questions, enter a code sent to her mobile phone number, or check her email to reset her password

Answers will vary.

Activity #1

Directions: Figure 2-1 presents a sample login page for a patient portal. Review the information and provide the **best** answer for the questions that follow.

1. Which of the following helps the system supporting the patient portal know who you are?

   A) Insurance policy number
   B) Date of birth
   (C) Username
   D) Password

2. Why would a user click on the "eye" icon when logging in to the portal?

   A) To reset their password

   B) To see the password they are typing ✓

   C) To check the number of characters in their password

   D) To see how strong their password is

3. Kameron wants online access to his health records. He has never used his patient portal before. What should he do to get started?

   A) Type his email address in the username field

   B) Log in

   C) Click the "Forgot Username" link

   D) Sign up ✓

4. Sandra can't remember her password and clicks on the "Forgot Password" link. What is most likely to happen next?

   A) She will be asked to call a support number for help.

   B) She will be asked to check her email to reset her password. ✓

   C) She will be asked to create a new account.

   D) None of the above

5. Why would a user choose the "pay as guest" option?

   A) They don't have an account yet, but need to pay a bill quickly.

   B) They only need to make a one-time payment and don't plan to use the portal often.

   C) They are helping a family member pay a bill.

   D) All of the above ✓

Activity #2

Directions: Look closely at **Figure 2-3**. The numbers in the picture point to different parts of the patient portal and what they do. Read each question carefully and circle the answer that best matches what you see in the picture and what you've learned about using a patient portal.

1. Which labels shows where to find the date of your next doctor's visit?

   A) Label 2   B) Label 3   C) Label 7 ✓

2. Where can you check if you have a bill from your last doctor's visit?

   A) Label 1   B) Label 11 ✓   C) Label 12

3. Which label shows where to change your password?

    A) Label 2   B) Label 4   **(C) Labels 4 and 6**

    Explanation: Both labels 4 and 6 will allow you to access the account settings and change information related to your account.

4. Which label shows where to click to log out of the patient portal?

    A) Label 1   **(B) Label 5**   C) Label 6

5. Where can you find a full list of menu options?

    (A) Label 1   B) Label 6   C) Label 12

6. Which label lets you change the language to Spanish?

    (A) Label 3   B) Label 4   C) Label 6

7. Which label shows the trends from your last 5 lab tests?

    A) Label 4   B) Label 8   **(C) Label 9**

8. Where do you go to send a private message about your health to your doctor?

    A) Label 1   B) Label 4   **(C) Label 8**

9. Which label allows you to view your main dashboard? *Note:* The **main dashboard** presents important information in one place and is the first page you see after you log in.

    A) Label 1   **(B) Label 2**   C) Labels 5

10. Which label takes you to your list of prescriptions or medicines?

    A) Label 4   B) Label 9   **(C) Label 10**

11. Where do you go to let a trusted family member or caregiver see your health information in the patient portal?

    (A) Label 4   B) Label 8   C) Label 12

12. Which label takes you to videos and articles your doctor thinks will help you stay healthy?

    A) Label 3   B) Label 8   **(C) Label 12**

Activity #3

Directions: In this lesson, you learned how patient portals can help you stay on track with preventive care. The activity below shows common health screenings for older adults. Draw a line to match each screening with the reason it helps individuals stay healthy.

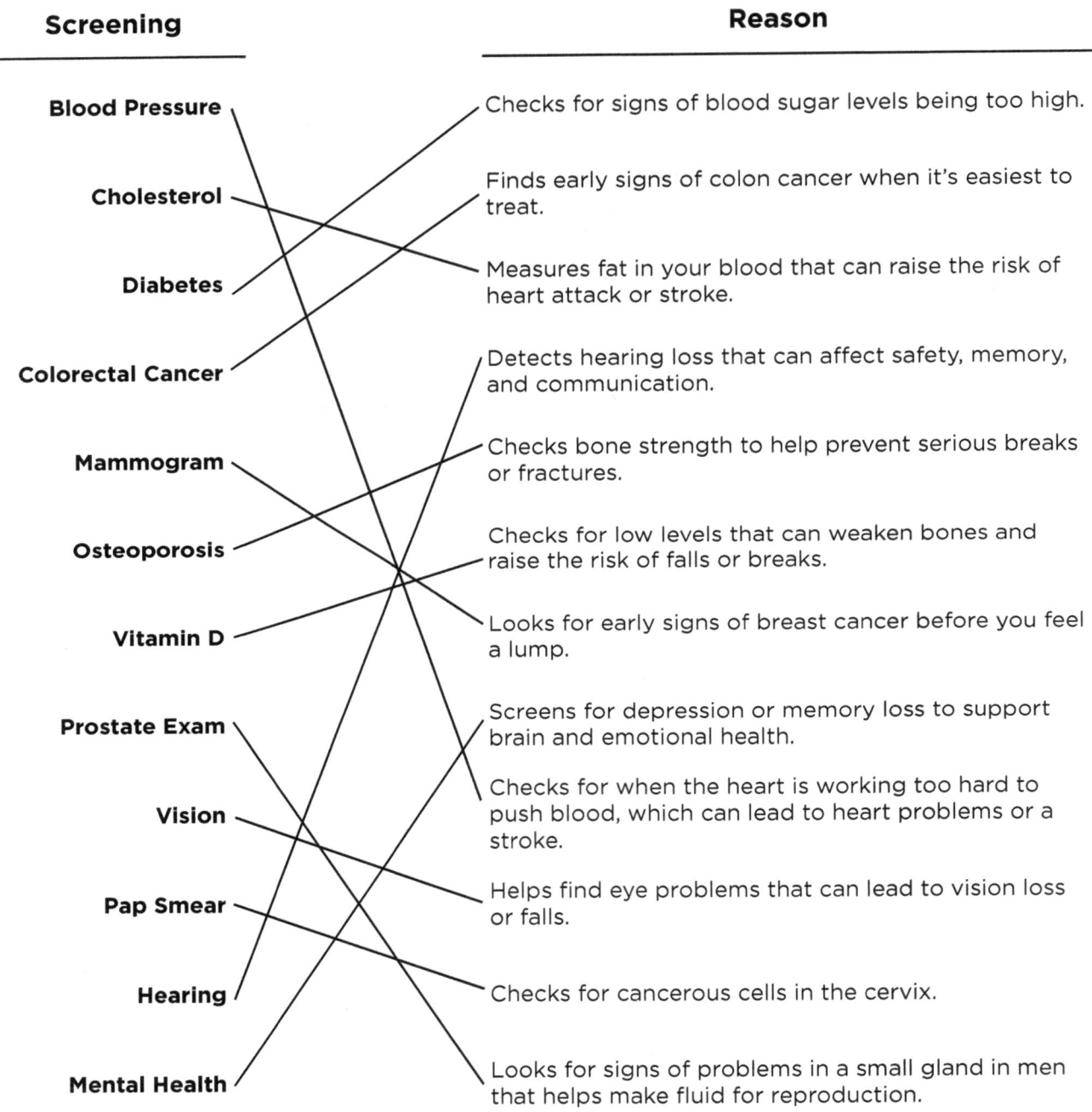

ANSWERS — LESSON THREE: Telehealth Visits

Activity #1

Directions: Read each question and provide the **best** answer.

1. Which of the following is a benefit of booking a doctor's appointment online?
    A) You have to wait on hold to talk to someone.
    (B) You can see available options and choose a time that works best for you.
    C) You must email staff to confirm the doctor's availability.
    D) You need to list all your symptoms before scheduling an appointment.

2. How is a doctor's visit for an *established patient* likely different from a *new patient*?
    A) A new patient pays less for their first visit.
    B) A new patient gets to go to the front of the line with no waiting.
    (C) An established patient may not need to fill out as many forms.
    D) An established patient always sees a different doctor.

3. Why is it necessary to select a provider before choosing a date and time?
    A) So the system knows your favorite doctor.
    B) So you can see how long the visit will take.
    C) So the doctor can match their schedule with your availability.
    (D) So the system can match you with the doctor's available times.

4. During the online scheduling process, why is the patient asked if they have seen their provider in the last 3 years?
    A) To know if the patient remembers their last visit.
    (B) To decide if the patient is new or returning.
    C) To find out if the patient has moved.
    D) To see if the patience has updated insurance information.

    Explanation: The correct answer is B. Asking this question helps the system assign the correct appointment type and time slot.

5. **True** or **False**. Write **T** for True or **F** for False next to the statements below.
    __T__ a) When scheduling an appointment online, you can jump to a future month.

__T__ b) When booking an appointment online, you will need to enter personal

__F__ c) Patients who schedule a doctor's appointment online are more likely to miss their visit.

Explanation: This statement is false. Data shows that online scheduling of doctor's appointments reduces no-shows, as reminders and confirmations are automatically sent to patients.

__T__ d) You can use online scheduling anytime — day or night.

__F__ e) Karen reports taking vitamin B12 on a regular basis and this information is included in her electronic health record. Karen's use of vitamin B12 tablets is not considered protected health information.

Explanation: This statement is false. Because Karen voluntarily reports taking vitamin B12 and this information is recorded in her online health records by her healthcare provider, it is considered PHI under HIPAA.

The R.E.E.L.

Directions: Melissa wants to show Nate how to use AI to organize his thoughts and understand his health better. What AI prompts can Melissa and Nate develop together that will help him feel ready to talk about his care with his doctor?

Prompts:
1. "Help me write questions to ask my doctor about my high blood pressure and how to manage it."
2. "What should I ask my doctor about my high blood sugar and how it can affect my health?"
3. "Explain what it means if my creatinine is high and what I can do to manage it."
4. "What should I tell my doctor about how I've been feeling, so they understand my health better?"
5. "Can you help me list steps I can take before my next lab test to stay healthy?"

Answers will vary.

Activity #2

Directions: Read each question and provide the **best** answer.

1. **Fill in the Blank**. Before a telehealth visit it's a good idea to _____.
    A) organize your medicines
    B) write down concerns about your health ✓
    C) turn off your phone to avoid distractions
    D) jot down how many hours you slept the night before

2. **Fill in the Blank**. Generative AI is similar to having a smart helper that can write, draw, or explain things in response to a _____ that you enter.
    A) question
    B) prompt ✓
    C) idea
    D) problem

3. How might a doctor's office confirm your identity during a telehealth visit?
    A) They will ask you to show a photo ID on camera.
    B) They will ask for your date of birth.
    C) They will ask for your home address.
    D) All of the above. ✓

4. Pam is preparing for a scheduled telehealth visit with her doctor. She needs your help figuring out the best course of action to take in order to get ready. Correctly order each step from one (1) to five (5) with one being the first step and five being the last step.

Step	Order (1 to 5)
Click the link to enter the virtual waiting room	4
Test your device camera and microphone	3
Check In	5
Write down questions beforehand	1
Find a quiet, private space	2

Activity #3

Directions: Tom Jackson is about to check in for his telehealth visit. **Figure 3-1** presents a screenshot of the welcome screen used by Tom's doctor's office for telehealth check-ins. Review **Figure 3-1** and answer the questions that follow.

1. Which doctor is Tom visiting?

    A) Dr. Kingsley   B) Dr. Towns   C) Dr. Wyatt

2. What must Tom do in order to check in?

    A) Turn on his camera   B) Enter his last name   **C) Enter "Tom Jackson"**

3. When Tom's doctor appears, Tom can see and hear his doctor, but his doctor can't hear him. What is the best thing Tom can do to fix the problem?

    A) Click the link in the appointment reminder email
    B) Check his audio settings
    C) Switch to a different browser

4. Five minutes into the virtual visit, Tom's video freezes. What is the best thing Tom can do to fix the problem?

    A) Leave the visit and call his doctor's office
    B) Turn off his camera and hope it starts working again
    C) Check his internet connection and try to reconnect

ANSWERS — LESSON FOUR: Everyday Care

Activity #1

Directions: Sara is using the Sugaroo™ app on her smartphone to help her think about how much sugar she is putting into her body. The app allows her to scan the barcode of her favorite foods and beverages and match the number of sugar cubes included in a serving for each item that she scans. One sugar cube equals roughly 4 grams of sugar.

Review the information and help Sara match the correct number of sugar cubes with her favorite beverages, by writing the letter of the sugar cube picture under the drink that it matches. Then, answer the questions that follow.

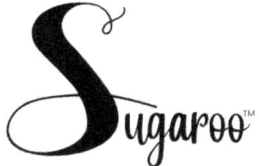

Daily Recommended Amount Sugar Cubes

A	B	C	D
E	F	G	H

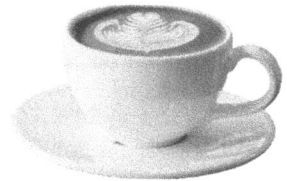

Cappuccino
(12 grams) __A__

Cranberry Juice
(48 Grams) __F__

Energy Drink
(56 grams) __H__

Sports Beverage
(56 grams) __H__

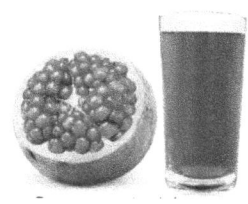

Pomegranate Juice
(36 grams) __C__

Root Beer
(44 Grams) __E__

Soda
(48 grams) __F__

Orange Juice
(40 grams) __D__

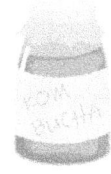

Kombucha
(28 grams) __B__

Note: **Kombucha** is a fizzy drink made from tea and natural good bacteria that can help with digestion. Sugar content in beverages based on data from Avera Health and Global News.[2,3]

Questions:

1. Check the statements that are true.

   ✓ Sara's favorite drinks, like soda and even fruit juice, add a lot of extra sugar to her diet.

   ✓ If Sara drinks any two of her favorite beverages in the same day, she exceeds the daily recommended amount of sugar.

   ___ Drinking kombucha will allow Sara to stay below the recommended daily amount of sugar.

   ✓ Drinking a cappuccino will allow Sara to stay below the recommended daily amount of sugar.

   ___ Based on the number of sugar cubes in her favorite drinks, Sara is putting very little sugar into her body.

   ✓ If Sara keeps drinking her favorite sugary drinks often, she could increase her risk of getting diabetes over time.

2. What are some other drinks Sara can choose to help her cut down on sugar?

   water, sparkling water, unsweetened iced tea, low-sugar sports drinks

   Answers will vary.

3. Based on the Sugaroo™ app, which of Sara's favorite drinks would you work to remove from your diet?

   Answers will vary.

Activity #2

Directions: Read each question and provide the **best** answer.

1. What is the primary purpose of remote patient monitoring?

   A) To find top-rated local clinics
   B) To communicate with your care team
   C) To track weight loss
   (D) To track health signs and share them with your doctor

2. Which of the following is *not* a vital sign that is usually checked during remote patient monitoring?
    A) Blood pressure
    B) Oxygen level
    C) Eye color
    D) Heart rate

3. Why is it helpful to send your health data to your doctor between visits?
    A) It replaces the need for future appointments.
    B) It helps the doctor better understand your health and choose the right treatment plan.
    C) It saves you time and money.
    D) The quality of care is better than in-person visits.

4. What can a body temperature of 101°F (38.3°C) tell your doctor?
    A) You are drinking enough water.
    B) You may have an infection.
    C) You need more sleep.
    D) You are hungry.

5. Why is it helpful to know your respiratory rate?
    A) To check if you're breathing normally
    B) To help count your daily steps
    C) To track your eating habits
    D) To improve your eyesight

6. What is a Patient-Reported Outcome (PRO)?
    A) A lab result
    B) A number from your smartwatch
    C) A message from your doctor
    D) How you say you feel

7. Which of the following shows a good PRO report?
    A) "I'm very dizzy and confused."
    B) "I didn't take my medicine this week."
    C) "No pain today. I walked 20 minutes."
    D) "I skipped breakfast and lunch."

8. **True** or **False**. Write **T** for True or **F** for False next to the statements below.

   __F__ a) A normal resting heart rate is the same for everyone.

   Explanation: This statement is false. Heart rate can vary by age, fitness, and health conditions.

   __T__ b) If your PRO report says "feeling tired all day" for many days in a row, your care team should know.

   Explanation: This statement is true. Knowing this information helps the care team check for issues and provide better support.

The R.E.E.L.

Directions: Imagine you want to stay in your home as you get older. If it makes sense for your health and finances, you'll need your circle of care (remember Lesson One) — and some helpful tools — to keep you safe, healthy, and connected.

Consider each situation and circle the "Care Help" that best applies to you.

Situation	Care Help (Circle all that apply, or write your own under "Other")			
1) You want reminders to take your medicine every day.	A. Care Coordinator	B. Family	C. Mobile Health App	D. Other _____
2) You feel sad and lonely and want someone to talk to.	A. Friend	B. Therapist	C. Community Health Worker	D. Other _____
3) You don't understand your lab results in the patient portal.	A. Care Coordinator	B. Nurse	C. AI Tool like ChatGPT	D. Other _____

Circle a tool below that you currently use or would consider using. Explain how it could help you or someone you know stay independent.

Patient Portal   Video Visits   Mobile Apps   Smartwatch   AI Chatbot

Answers will vary to all of the above.

ANSWERS — LESSON FIVE: Trusting Health Information

Activity #1

Directions: Read each scenario and identify the emotional trigger as either cognitive bias, propaganda, or fear. Circle the **best** answer.

1. Heather reads the following social media ad: *"Join the wellness revolution now! Everyone is doing it — don't be left out."* Heather doesn't want to miss out so she signs up and becomes a member.

    Cognitive Bias   (**Propaganda**)   Fear

2. Martin believes a certain herbal tea cures colds, so he only reads articles and watches videos that say it works, while ignoring research showing no benefit.

    (**Cognitive Bias**)   Propaganda   Fear

3. Eddie and Sam are miners who work in underground tunnels. Sam goes to a local sauna each week and wants Eddie to join him. He says the following to Eddie: "If you don't detox soon, your body will be full of dangerous toxins."

    Cognitive Bias   Propaganda   (**Fear**)

4. After hearing about a rare side effect from a friend's mammogram, Michelle believes it's common, even though data shows it almost never happens. She decides to cancel her upcoming appointment and reschedule it for next year.

    (**Cognitive Bias**)   Propaganda   Fear

5. As Kyle prepares to watch his favorite podcast, he sees an ad that claims that eating a certain food will ruin his health forever. It just so happens that Kyle eats this food on a regular basis and decides to click the link to learn more.

    Cognitive Bias   Propaganda   (**Fear**)

6. Beverly wants to get healthier and has a goal of losing at least 20 pounds. She hears her favorite talk show host talk about a certain diet that "guarantees" fast results. This claim stays in her mind, even after her doctor explains there is no proof it works. Beverly decides to try the diet anyway.

    (**Cognitive Bias**)   Propaganda   Fear

7. Travis went to his local clinic after hurting his knee. The waiting room was full because many people were being treated for overdoses from a "bad batch" of **opioid drugs** (strong painkillers that can be very addictive). The next day on the news, a politician said the City's drug problem was under control and there was no reason to worry.

    Cognitive Bias   (**Propaganda**)   Fear

8. Sergio has type 2 diabetes and sees this online ad described in the photo. He carefully considers purchasing the "breakthrough pill" for himself.

   Cognitive Bias   (Propaganda)   Fear

9. What is the reason for your choice in Scenario #8?

   The scenario uses over-the-top, attention-grabbing words like "breakthrough," "reverses diabetes," and "just 10 days" to create excitement and make people believe it, without giving any proof. This kind of language is a sign of propaganda.

   Answers will vary.

Activity #2

Directions: Read each question and provide the **best** answer.

1. Identify all the trigger words, or phrases, in the following advertisement.

   "Erase every wrinkle instantly with our miracle injection! Look 20 years younger in just one week — guaranteed. Unlike anything you've ever seen, this perfect treatment gives you flawless, youthful skin that lasts forever. Everyone will notice your transformation, and you'll never feel old again."

   erase, instantly, miracle, 20 years younger, guaranteed, perfect, flawless, lasts forever, everyone, never

2. **Microplastics** are tiny pieces of plastic that break down from bottles, bags, and other plastic products. They are so small you usually can't see them, but they can end up in food, water, and even the air.[10]

   A well-known online influencer makes a claim about microplastics, as shown below. Identify all the trigger words, or phrases, that sound extreme or designed to scare you.

   "Everyone who drinks bottled water is filling their body with deadly microplastics! These tiny plastic pieces, smaller than a grain of sand, are invading your organs and causing cancer in millions of people. No one is safe — every sip adds poison to your system. Stop drinking bottled water now, before it's too late!"

   everyone, deadly, invading, millions, no one is safe, poison, before it's too late

3. Review the words you identified in the first two questions. How do they make

the claims more emotional than factual?

> The trigger words stir feelings instead of providing real facts.

Answers will vary.

4. What real evidence would you need to check before believing either claim?

> Check if trusted studies or medical experts have tested them and shared results. Look for data from reliable sources like health organizations, peer-reviewed research, or government health sites. If a claim cannot show clear evidence, it is likely misleading or exaggerated.

Answers will vary.

5. Norman's doctor tells him that his blood pressure is very high and provides a treatment plan, which includes medication, cutting back on salty foods, and walking 20 minutes each day. Norman shares the news with his wife and tells her that given his luck, he will "probably have a stroke tomorrow."

Apply the CLEAR Framework (CLEAR Head Approach) to help Norman make smart choices with a calm, clear mind.

C	a) How can Norman cool his feelings? He can take a few deep breaths and remind himself that fear can make things feel worse than they are.
L	b) What trigger words did Norman use to jump to the worst possible outcome? "probably" and "tomorrow"
E	c) How can Norman envision a positive health outcome? Instead of picturing a stroke tomorrow, he can envision lowering his blood pressure over time and being healthy enough to enjoy his family and activities.
A	d) How can Norman attend to what he can control? He can follow his doctor's treatment plan and take his medication, cut back on salty foods, and walk for 20 minutes each day.
R	e) What can Norman do if his mind jumps to worst case thinking? He can repeat CLEAR to bring his focus back to what he can do now.

The R.E.E.L.

Scenario: Joel is a medical assistant who works at a local clinic. He sees patients with low literacy, vision problems, and limited typing skills. He wants to know how encouraging the use of voice tools for AI fact-finding can lead to more meaningful, two-way conversations with these patients.

Based on your knowledge, what response will you share with Joel?

Using voice tools can make it easier for patients who struggle with reading, writing, or typing. Instead of getting stuck on spelling or small screens, they can simply ask questions out loud. This helps them focus on what they really want to know.

When patients can speak their questions, they are more likely to share their concerns openly. This gives providers a chance to listen, respond, and guide them toward safe, trustworthy information.

Answers will vary.

Activity #3

Directions: Read each scenario and write an AI fact-finding prompt (question you would ask) to help make sense of the situation.

Scenario 1: Vicky and Sam's Son Zack

Vicky and Sam's son, Zack, is in first grade. His teacher says Zack has a hard time finishing his work and paying attention. He also has trouble sitting still in class. The school nurse thinks it could be ADHD and even mentions that Zack might need medicine called a stimulant. She reminds them to see a doctor for a second opinion. Before the appointment, Vicky and Sam want to use AI to look up facts so they can ask better questions and understand what's really going on.

What is ADHD in young children, how is it usually diagnosed, and what do parents need to know about stimulant medicines? Please explain in plain language and suggest some questions we can ask the doctor.

Answers will vary.

Scenario 2: Understanding a Measles Outbreak

Natasha lives in a small rural county. Recently, there has been a measles outbreak affecting her community and a region of roughly 650,000 people. So far, there have been 700 cases, 100 hospitalizations, and 2 deaths. The local news is reporting on the outbreak nonstop, and it feels overwhelming. Natasha wants to use AI to make sense of the numbers so she can understand how serious the outbreak is and come up with better questions to ask her doctor or public health officials.

> Help me understand a measles outbreak in a region of about 650,000 people. There are 700 cases, 100 hospitalizations, and 2 deaths. Explain what these numbers mean in simple terms, how serious this is, and what questions I should ask my doctor or local health officials.

Answers will vary.

Scenario 3: Reading Food Labels

Tyrone is looking at the label on one of his favorite snack foods. He sees that the ingredients list includes monosodium glutamate (MSG) and some artificial colors called Yellow 6, Yellow 5, and Red 40. Tyrone isn't sure what these ingredients are or if they are safe to eat. He decides to use AI to look up reliable information so that he can ask better questions when he talks with a nutritionist.

> Explain in simple terms what monosodium glutamate (MSG), Yellow 5, Yellow 6, and Red 40 are. Tell me what they do in food, if they are safe to eat, and if there are any health concerns I should know about.

Answers will vary.

ANSWERS–LESSON SIX: Protecting Health Information

Activity #1

Directions: Read each question. Circle the **best** answer.

1. Which of the following is a right patients have under HIPAA?
    A) The right to have personal protective equipment (PPE) like KN95 masks in the waiting room for their use.
    B) The right to get a copy of their medical records and share them with someone they trust.
    C) The right to choose which staff member takes their blood pressure.
    D) The right to question the accuracy of a bill.

2. Which of the following is an example of how HIPAA protects patient privacy?

    A) A hospital lets a patient choose the time they would like to bathe.
    B) A patient is told they can't eat or drink before a surgery.
    C) A nurse explains to a patient that their lab results will only be shared with doctors involved in their care.
    D) A clinic posts everyone's test results on a bulletin board so staff can see them.

3. Which of the following is not an example of care operations?

    A) Training staff on how to grow in their jobs or move into new roles.
    B) Reviewing charts to make sure treatments are safe and follow best practices.
    C) Looking at data to find ways to shorten wait times or improve patient care.
    D) Checking patient records to see if people are getting needed screenings.

4. Jamal notices his medical record says he is allergic to penicillin, but he is not. He asks the clinic to correct it. Which right is Jamal exercising?

    A) Right to See His Records
    B) Right to Fix Mistakes
    C) Right to Know How His Information is Used
    D) Right to Ask for Limits

5. Freddie tells his doctor not to share information about his therapy sessions with his insurance company. The doctor listens, but explains they may not always be able to agree. Which right is Freddie using?

    A) Right to See His Records
    B) Right to Fix Mistakes
    C) Right to Know How His Information is Used
    D) Right to Ask for Limits

6. Before her first visit, Gloria receives a paper that explains how the clinic may share her health information. Which right is Gloria using?

    A) Right to See Her Records
    B) Right to Fix Mistakes
    C) Right to Know How Her Information is Used
    D) Right to Ask for Limits

7. Teresa asks her clinic for a copy of her lab results so she can bring them to a specialist. Which right is Teresa asking for?
   - **A) Right to See Her Records** ✓
   - B) Right to Fix Mistakes
   - C) Right to Know How Her Information is Used
   - D) Right to Ask for Limits

8. Tom sees that his medical record says he takes a weight-loss drug, but he has never been prescribed it, so he asks to have it corrected. Which right is Tom asking for?
   - A) Right to See His Records
   - **B) Right to Fix Mistakes** ✓
   - C) Right to Know How His Information is Used
   - D) Right to Ask for Limits

Patient Responsibilities

Questions: Consider the following two emails. Can you tell which one is safe and which one is a scam? What red flags appear in the scam email?

Figure 6-2 is the safe email and Figure 6-1 is the scam email. Red flags in the scam email include an urgent tone, threat of care being delayed, and a strange link asking for a password.

Answers will vary.

Activity #2

Directions: Read each question. Provide the **best** answer(s).

1. The table below contains twelve (12) potential passwords. Circle the **strong** passwords using the information you have learned about features of a good password.

987654321=	Password7	**!25Dwq83Pfn** ✓	batman
bw?39P7dxp ✓	flower	football	Trustno1
dragon	**mZ26=f391B** ✓	princess	**s94U$G593h** ✓

2. What does two-factor authentication (2FA) mean?

   A) Using two different doctors to confirm a **diagnosis,** which is the name for a health problem.

   B) Writing your password down in two places.

   C) Logging in twice to make sure your account is safe.

   (D) Logging in with a password plus a second step, like a code.

3. Why is two-factor authentication safer than just a password?

   A) It makes logging in faster.

   B) It only works on mobile phones.

   (C) It adds another layer of security if your password is stolen.

   D) It hides your password from your care team.

4. Judith is logging in to the online account provided by her health clinic. She receives a six digit code in her email and enters it. What should Judith do next? (Use **Figure 6-3** as a reference.)

   A) Click the "Send New Code" button.

   (B) Click the "Submit" button.

   C) Go back to the previous page.

   D) Contact customer care.

5. Jorge is logging in to the online account provided by his health clinic. He receives a six digit code in his email, but he can't remember his email password. What should Jorge do next? (Use **Figure 6-3** as a reference.)

   A) Call his doctor and ask for the code over the phone.

   B) Keep guessing passwords until he gets into his email.

   (C) Contact customer care.

   D) Ask a friend to log in to his email instead.

   Explanation: Per Figure 6-3, Jorge should contact customer care. Alternatively, he can use the "Forgot Password" option to reset his email password so he can get the code.

Activity #3

Directions: Read each scenario. Then, write what should have been done differently, if anything, to keep the patient's information safe and private, and avoid a HIPAA violation.

1. **Sharing Without Permission.** A surgery clinic gave a patient's private health information to a research group without asking the patient first or getting approval from a review board.

   They should have asked the patient to sign a consent form or received special approval from a privacy board before sharing information.

   Answers will vary.

2. **Withholding Records.** A doctor's office refused to give a patient their medical records because the patient still owed money.

   Patients must be allowed to see their records, even if they owe money. The office should have provided the records.

   Answers will vary.

3. **Calling a Patient's Name.** A nurse calls out, "Miguel Lopez?" in the waiting room to bring him back for his appointment.

   This is okay under HIPAA because staff are allowed to use patient names as part of normal care.

   Answers will vary.

4. **Unnecessary Sharing.** A hospital emailed an Operating Room schedule to staff that included details about an employee's surgery, which their supervisor (not part of the treatment team) could see.

   The hospital should only share patient information with staff directly involved in the patient's care, not with supervisors or others.

   Answers will vary.

5. **Labels That Expose.** A dental office put a red sticker that said "No COVID Vaccine" on some patient charts, where anyone could see it.

   The dental office should keep sensitive health details inside the chart or in a secure system, not on visible stickers.

   Answers will vary.

6. **Family Member at the Visit.** A patient brings her husband into the exam room. The doctor talks about her diagnosis with both of them present.

   This is okay under HIPAA because the patient gave permission by inviting her husband into the room..

   Answers will vary.

7. **No Privacy Notice.** A mental health center did not give a father and his daughter (the patient) a written notice explaining how the daughter's health information would be used before her evaluation.

   The center should have given the father and daughter a "Notice of Privacy Practices" before the evaluation, explaining their rights and how information is used.

   Answers will vary.

ANSWERS—LESSON SEVEN: Working with Your Care Team

Activity #1

Directions: Read each scenario. Refer to **Figure 7-2** to describe the positive outcome.

1. Tammy notices swelling in her ankles and messages her doctor through the patient portal. Her care team adjusts her medicine right away, and she avoids kidney failure.

   By getting help early, Tammy stays healthier and avoids emergency care.

   Answers will vary.

2. Paul goes to his yearly checkup and gets a cancer screening. The test finds a small problem early, and it is treated before it gets worse.

   Paul's cancer screening helped his care team find a small problem early and treat it before it turned into something more serious.

   Answers will vary.

3. Mr. Grant takes his blood pressure medicine every day as prescribed. At his next checkup, his blood pressure is under control, and he no longer feels dizzy.

   Mr. Grant takes his medicine as directed. As a result, he feels better and avoids serious health problems.

   Answers will vary.

4. Ms. Alvarez struggles to get healthy food because she doesn't drive. Her clinic connects her with a local food delivery program. With better meals and exercise, her diabetes is under control.

   Ms. Alvarez receives support for a social need like food. She is now calmer, has more energy, and can better manage her diabetes.

   Answers will vary.

5. Rosa uses a health app to track her blood sugar and notice which foods make it go up or down. By changing what she eats and sharing the numbers with her nurse, her blood sugar improves and she moves from diabetic to pre-diabetic.

   Rosa tracks her blood sugar levels and food. As a result, her blood sugar improves, and her risk for problems goes down.

   Answers will vary.

Activity #2
Practice Survey: How Was Your Care Experience?

Directions – Part A: Think back to a recent visit with a doctor, nurse, or health worker — either in person or by phone/video. This survey helps you think about what worked well and where things could improve. Circle the answer that best matches your experience.

Answers will vary.

The R.E.E.L.

The following story is about an 81-year-old woman who followed her doctor's orders and used AI to learn more about her health, but was afraid to speak up.

Directions: Read each step in Debbie's story. At each step, decide if it shows Strong Partnership or a Missed Opportunity. Circle your choice and answer the reflection questions that follow.

Step 1 – First Visit

Debbie, age 81, develops a skin rash she's never had before. She tells her doctor, who sends her to an **allergist** (a doctor who tests and treats people for allergies, like reactions to food, pollen, or medicine). The allergy tests come back negative.

(Strong Partnership)   Missed Opportunity

Step 2 – Using AI

Debbie describes her symptoms to an AI tool. The AI suggests the correct diagnosis and treatment: an oral medicine plus a **topical cream** (a medicine you rub on your skin to treat a problem in that area). Debbie's daughter does similar research and encourages her to ask the doctor about the oral medicine.

(Strong Partnership)   Missed Opportunity

Step 3 – Dermatologist Visit

Debbie's doctor refers her to a **dermatologist** (a doctor who treats problems with the skin, hair, and nails). The dermatologist prescribes only the cream. Debbie does not mention what the AI suggested, and her daughter confirmed, about the oral medicine.

Strong Partnership   **(Missed Opportunity)**

Step 4 – Follow-Up

At her follow-up visit, Debbie tells the dermatologist the rash is better but she still has itching. The dermatologist says she's fine and needs no more treatment.

Strong Partnership   **(Missed Opportunity)**

Step 5 – Outcome

Two weeks later, the rash comes back. Debbie realizes the **mites** (tiny bugs that can lay eggs under the skin and cause itching and rashes) are still in her system. She wishes she had spoken up about what the AI suggested.

Strong Partnership   **(Missed Opportunity)**

Reflection Questions:

1. What could have changed if Debbie had shared the AI's suggestion with her dermatologist?

   The dermatologist might have looked into the oral medicine and treated the problem fully, not just the rash on her skin.

   Answers will vary.

2. Why is it important for patients to speak up, even if they think the doctor knows more?

   Doctors have knowledge, but patients know their bodies and experiences best. Sharing everything helps the care team make better decisions.

   Answers will vary.

3. How can staff encourage patients like Debbie to share what they learn from digital tools?

   Staff can ask questions like, "Have you looked up anything about your symptoms?" or "Is there anything else you've learned that you'd like me to know?"

   Answers will vary.